JUICING BIBLE FOR WEIGHT LOSS

50 Recipes to Total Detox, Reboot, Feel Young, Live Longer and to Prevent Diseases

7 Day Detox Juicing and 5 Day Juicing Reboot Plans

DISCLAIMER

Losing weight is not that easy after all. Tasteless salads, vigorous workouts and avoiding the temptation to eat your favorite food…these are all part of a standard weight loss plan. And these are the things that make it boring and difficult to lose weight. So how about something much more interesting and easier?

Well, we are talking about juice diets. Everybody likes fruits and vegetable juices and smoothies. What if we say that you can actually lose weight and detoxify your body with these drinks? This is what this book is all about. It is unlike any other boring recipe tome containing tasteless and bland recipes.

Healthy, refreshing, energetic and most importantly delicious – This is what the "*Juicing Bible of Weight Loss*" is all about. It contains the following.

1. More than 50 different juice reboot and detoxification recipes.

2. Serving size and cooking time of each recipe.

3. Nutritional facts with each recipe. Now this is something that you won't find in many juicing recipe books.

4. 5 – day Juicing reboot plan with recipes

5. 7 day Detox juicing plan with recipes

6. Images and collages to make the book more pleasing and colorful.

The recipes stated in this book are very easy with most of the ingredients mostly available in a standard kitchen pantry.

So don't just stop here. Try out a few recipes and feel young and refreshed like you have never before.

Table of Contents

ALL TIME DETOX DRINKS

Detox Dandelion Water

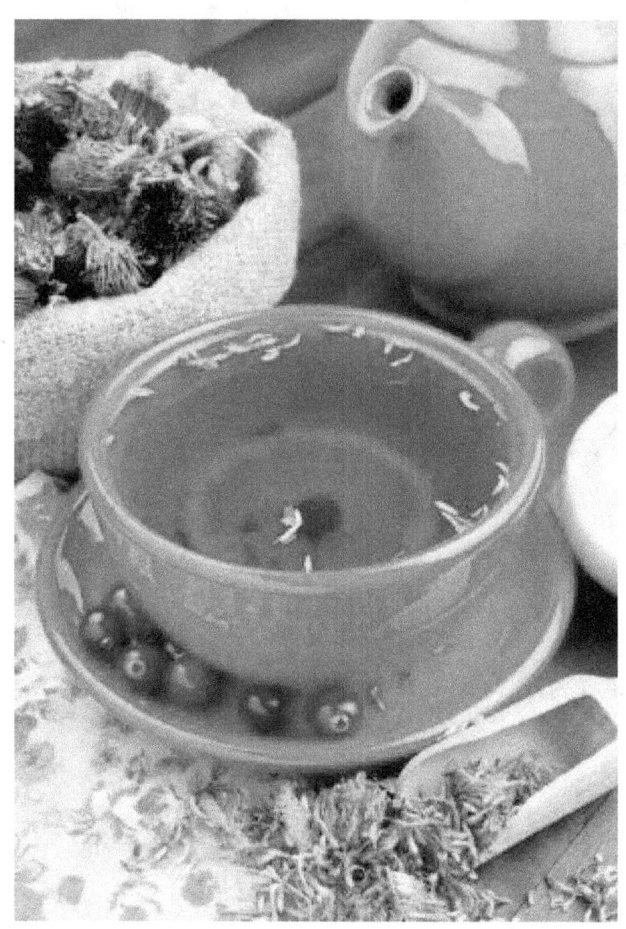

SERVES 1

Cooking Time: 2 minutes

Nutritional Facts: Calories 12, Total Fat 0 g, Protein 0.1 g, Carbohydrates 3.8 g

Ingredients

    2 Tbsp fresh lemon juice

    7 cups distilled water

    1 dandelion root tea bag

    1 Tbsp 100% pure cranberry juice

Preparation Method

Combine water, lemon juice and cranberry juice in a pitcher. Stir to mix.

Add the tea bag.

Drink it throughout the day while the tea bag is still in the pitcher.

Green Juicy Reboot

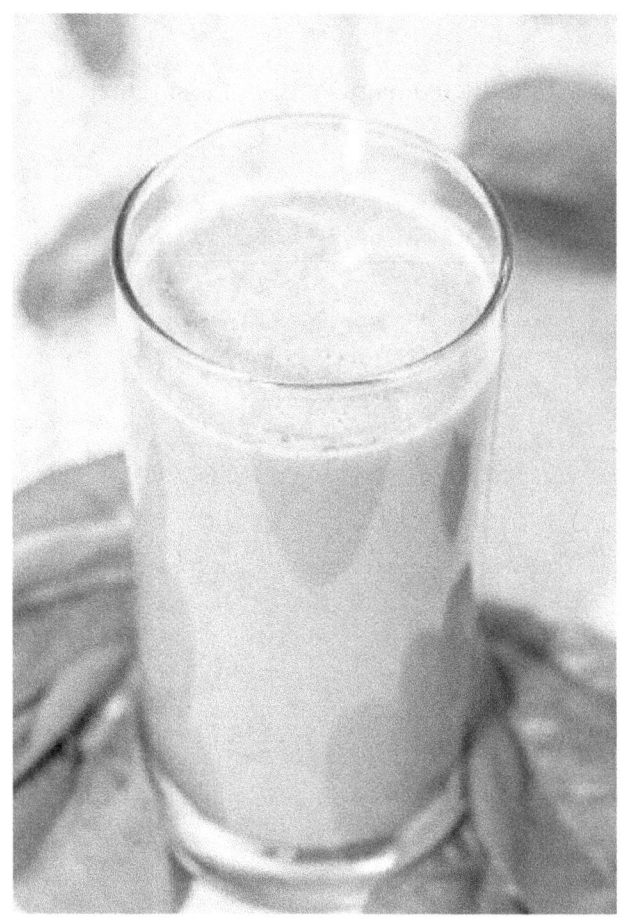

SERVES 4

Cooking Time: 3 minutes

Nutritional Facts: Calories 143, Protein 4.2 g, Total Fat 1.1 g, Carbohydrates 36 g

Ingredients

12 leaves of kale

4 green apples, cored and cut into halves

1 lemon, peeled

1 piece of fresh ginger (2 inch)

8 stalks of celery, remove the leaves

2 medium cucumbers

Preparation Method

Process all the ingredients in an electric blender till it becomes a smoothie.

Serve!

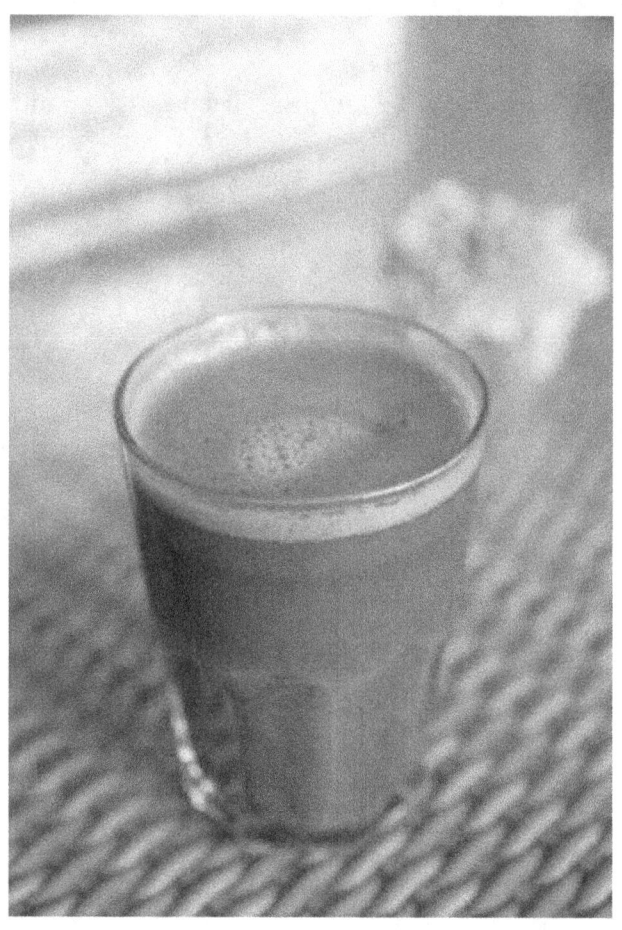

SERVES 2

Cooking Time: 5 minutes

Nutritional Facts: Calories 221, Protein 6.4 g, Total Fat 1.4 g, Carbohydrates 52 g

Ingredients

    4 large sized carrots, juiced

    24 long snap beans

    1 large apple, juiced

    2 small beets, juiced

    20 sprigs of parsley

    4 stalks of celery

    2 small cucumbers

Preparation Method

Process all the ingredients in a juicer.

Serve!

Kiwi Detox Juice

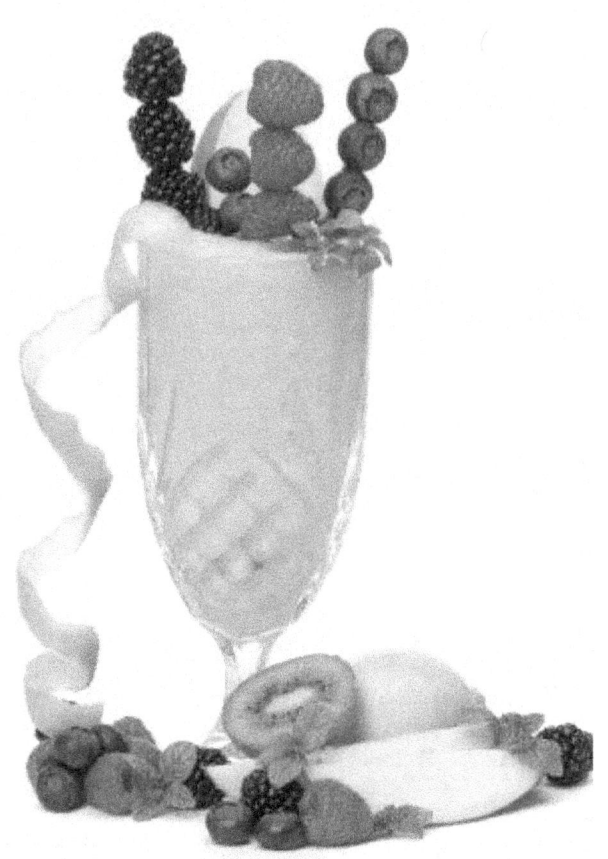

SERVES 2 – 3

Cooking Time: 3 minutes

Nutritional Facts: Calories 164, Protein 2.1 g, Total Fat 0.8 g, Carbohydrates 39.5 g

Ingredients

4 medium sized kiwifruit, peeled and coarsely diced

4 fresh mint leaves

1 cup diced mango

1 ½ cups fresh pineapple juice

Preparation Method

Combine all the ingredients in an electric blender.

Pulse till smooth.

Enjoy!

High-Fiber Red Blend

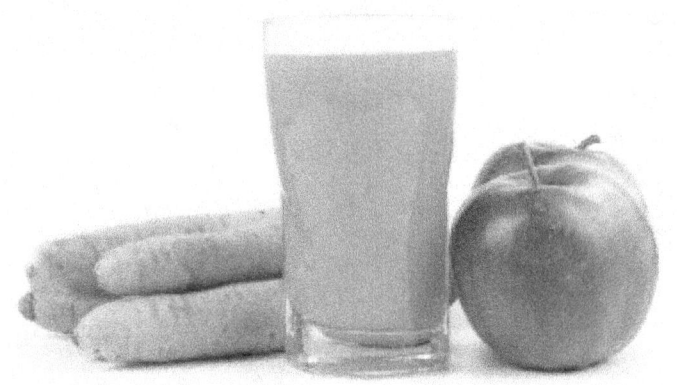

SERVES 2

Cooking Time: 2 hours

Nutritional Facts: Calories 155, Protein 3 g, Total Fat 0.7 g, Carbohydrates 37 g

Ingredients

>   1 medium sized apple, cored and cut into cubes
>
>   14 grams fresh ginger, peeled and chopped (about 2 Tbsp after chopping)
>
>   1 cup water
>
>   4 carrots, scrubbed and cut into slices
>
>   1 beet, peeled and coarsely chopped

Preparation Method

Combine all the ingredients in a blender.

Pulse till smooth, while stopping occasionally to scrape down the sides.

Pass the juice through a sieve.

Discard the residues and put the juice in the refrigerator for 2 hours.

Stir or shake well before serving.

Classic Detox Lemonade

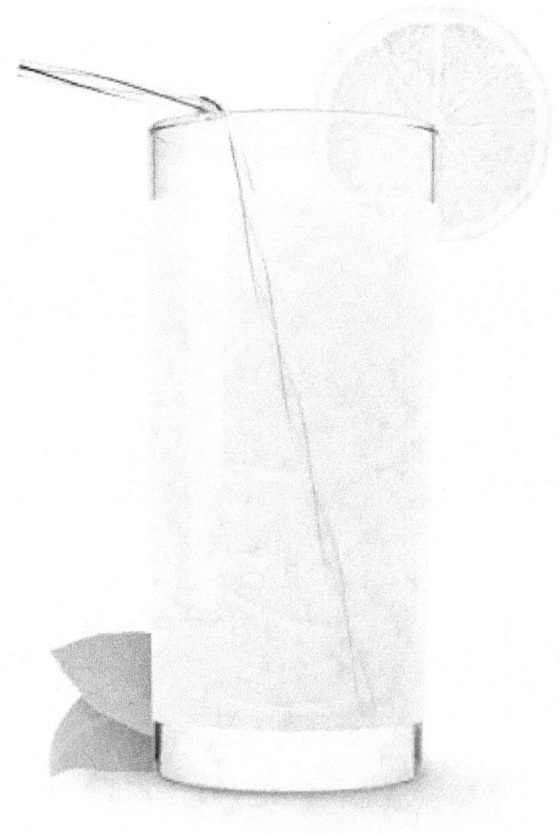

SERVES 5

Cooking Time: 5 minutes

Nutritional Facts: Calories 113, Protein 0.1 g, Total Fat 0.1 g, Carbohydrates 29.6 g

Ingredients

¾ cup Maple Syrup

5 cups water

½ tsp freshly ground black pepper

3 lemons, juiced

Preparation Method

Combine all the ingredients in a bottle.

Lid the bottle, shake and serve!

Fruit and Veggie Detox Smoothie

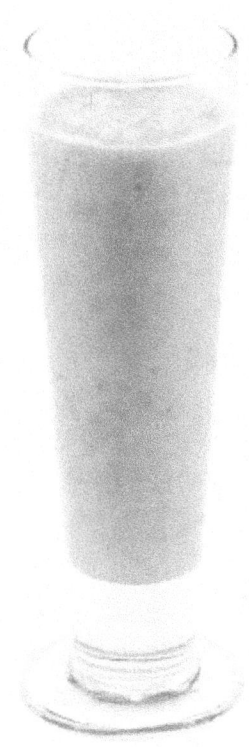

SERVES 2 – 3

Cooking Time: 5 minutes

Nutritional Facts: Calories 114, Protein 2 g, Total Fat 0.4 g, Carbohydrates 29 g

Ingredients

8 fl oz. water (about 1 ½ cup)

1 cup raw cilantro

1 medium sized pear

1 banana (about 7 inches long)

¼ cup chopped Celery

2 cups spinach

1 medium Apple, cored and cut into large chunks

1 lemon, juiced

¼ cup parsley

Preparation Method

Blend together all the ingredients.

Serve!

Detoxifying Orange Juice

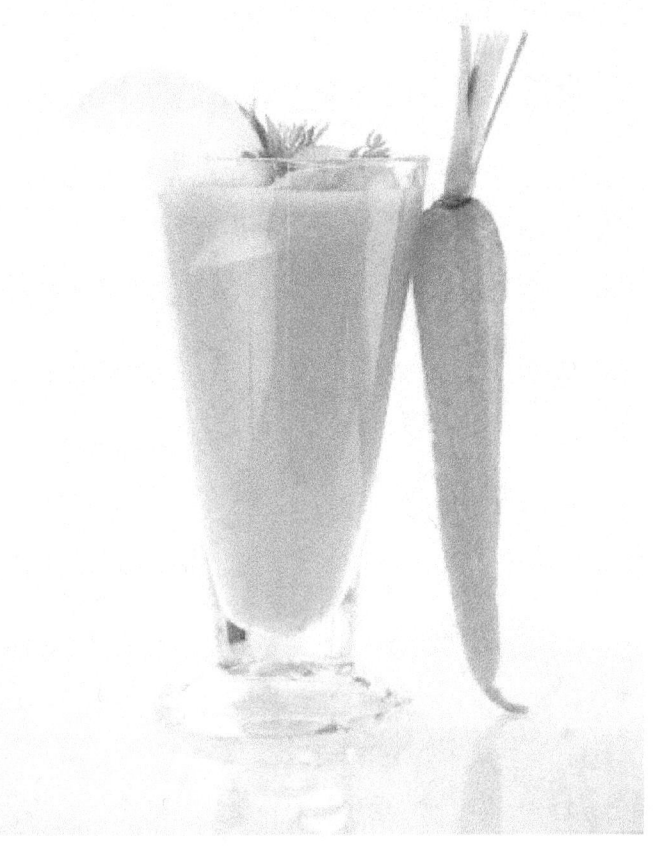

SERVES 4

Cooking Time: 10 – 15 minutes

Nutritional Facts: Calories 147, Protein 3.3 g, Total Fat 0.6 g, Carbohydrates 35.7 g

Ingredients

8 cloves of garlic, crushed

8 medium sized fresh carrots, peeled and juiced

4 slices ginger roots, crushed

260 ml water (a little over one cup)

5 oranges, juiced

Preparation Method

Combine water, ginger and garlic in a saucepan.

Bring it to a boil over medium flame.

Turn off the heat and allow it cool for a while.

Stir in the orange juice and carrot juice.

Whisk well and serve!

Chunky Red Juice Reboot

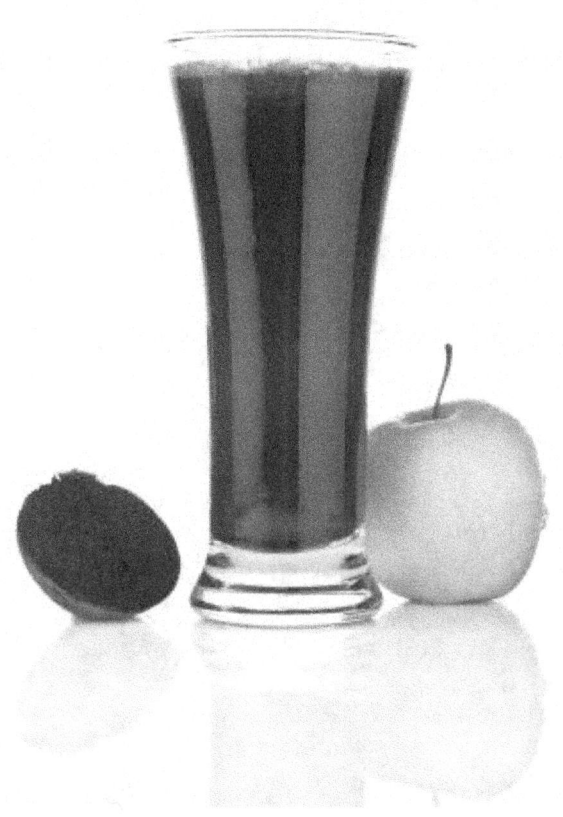

SERVES 2

Cooking Time: 3 minutes

Nutritional Facts: Calories 322, Protein 5.2 g, Total Fat 1.8 g, Carbohydrates 78.5 g

Ingredients

> 4 small sized beets, peeled and cut into large chunks
>
> 6 medium carrots, scrubbed and coarsely sliced
>
> 4 small apples, cored and coarsely cubed

Preparation Method

Process all the ingredients in a juicer.

Pulse till all the things are juiced, yet slightly chunky.

Drink immediately.

Herbilicious Apple Detox Drink

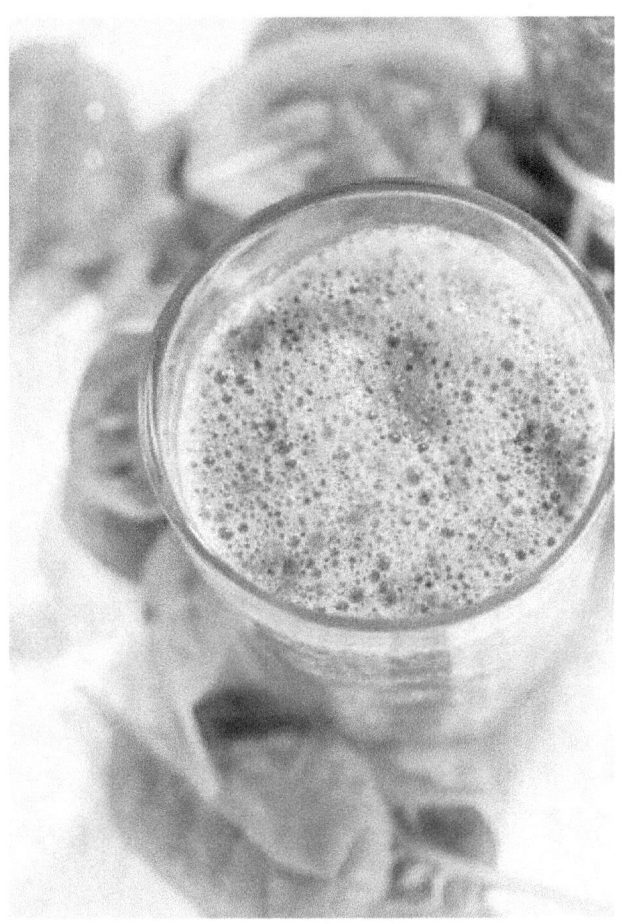

SERVES 6

Cooking Time: 4 – 5 minutes

Nutritional Facts: Calories 97.6, Protein 4.5 g, Total Fat 1 g, Carbohydrates 24 g

Ingredients

> 4 medium apples
>
> 2 bunches of celery
>
> 1 bunch of spinach or kale or romaine lettuce, washed and pat dry
>
> 1 (1-inch) piece of fresh ginger
>
> 1 bunch of chard or parsley, washed and pat dry
>
> 2 lemons, juiced

2 cucumbers

Preparation Method

Peel the cucumbers.

Core and cut the apples into large chunks.

Combine all the ingredients in a blender or juicer.

Pulse till it becomes a puree. Add water if you want to thin out its consistency.

Serve as it is or put it in the refrigerator to chill.

Enjoy!

Green Alkalinity Drink

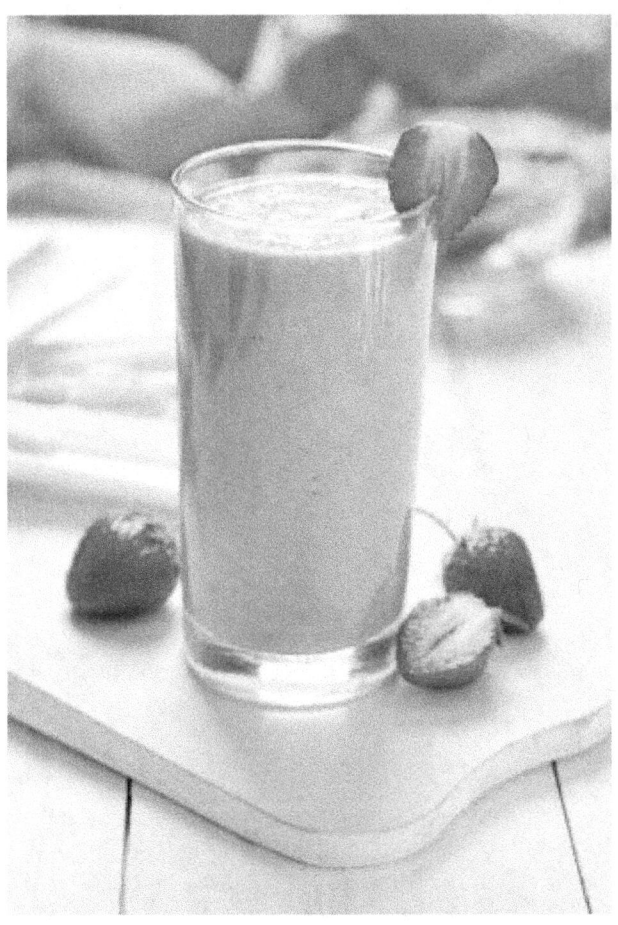

SERVES 4

Cooking Time: 3 – 4 minutes

Nutritional Facts: Calories 85, Protein 2.3 g, Total Fat 0.7 g, Carbohydrates 21 g

Ingredients

8 stalks of celery

2 medium pears, juiced

2 cups tightly packed raw kale

1 lime, juiced

1 piece of fresh ginger root (about 1 inch)

Preparation Method

Run all the ingredients through an electric juicer.

Put celery after kale to push the kale through the juicer.

Enjoy!

Herbs and Berries Juice

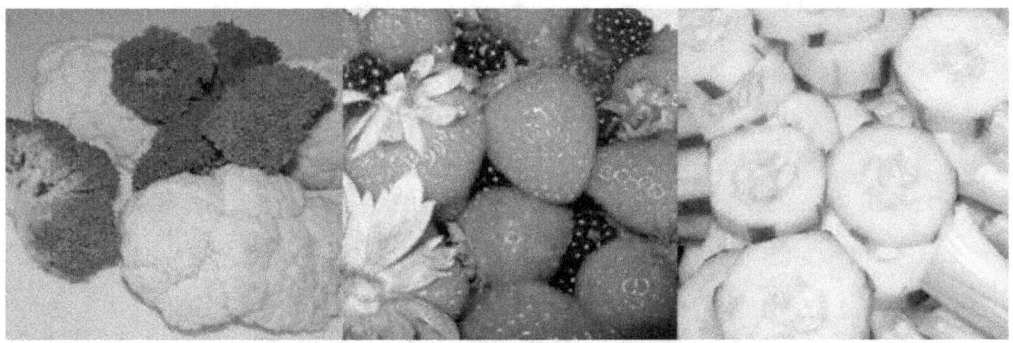

SERVES 4

Cooking Time: 4 – 5 minutes

Nutritional Facts: Calories 107.3, Protein 7 g, Total Fat 1.1 g, Carbohydrates 22.1 g

Ingredients

> 2 cups fresh broccoli
>
> 4 cups baby greens
>
> 4 medium sized red ripe tomatoes, coarsely diced
>
> 4 large leaves of kale
>
> 9 – 10 fresh strawberries, cut into halves
>
> 4 large leaves of Swiss Chard, washed and pat dry
>
> 2 cups coarsely chopped cauliflower
>
> 2 stalks of raw celery, washed and coarsely chopped
>
> Half cup fresh blueberries
>
> 1 medium cucumber, peel-on chopped

Preparation Method

Run all the ingredients through a masticating juicer (like Omega 8005).

Serve as it is or chilled!

Simple Beet Juicing Reboot

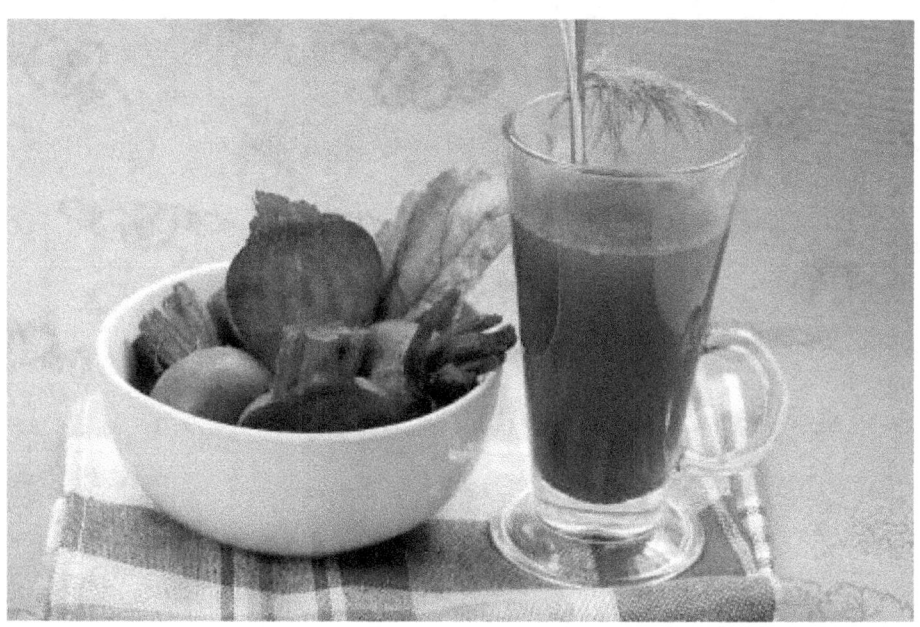

SERVES 2

Cooking Time: 3 minutes

Nutritional Facts: Calories 82.6, Protein 1.3 g, Total Fat 0.1 g, Carbohydrates 20 g

Ingredients

> 2 beets, washed and pat dry
>
> Half cup fresh mint sprigs

Preparation Method

Run the beets and mint through a juice extractor.

Serve!

Fruit and Veggie Detox Drink

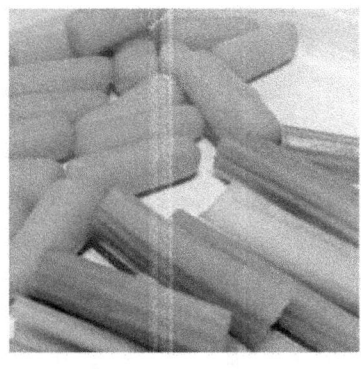 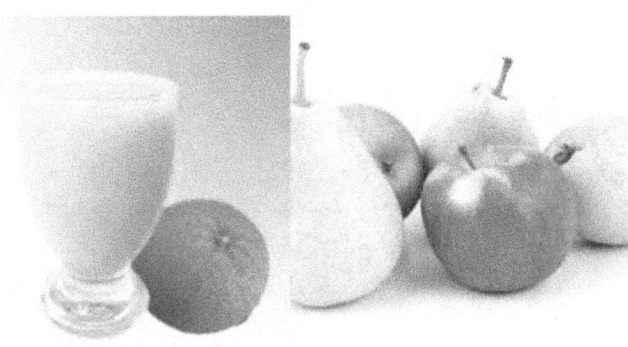

SERVES 2

Cooking Time: 5 minutes

Nutritional Facts: Calories 447, Protein 12.7 g, Total Fat 2.4 g, Carbohydrates 111 g

Ingredients

   2 pears, coarsely chopped

   2 medium tomatoes, coarsely chopped

   2 handfuls of kale

   2 oranges, juiced

   2 carrots, rinsed and coarsely sliced

   1 lemon, juiced

   4 stalks of celery, rinsed and coarsely chopped

   2 apples, cored and coarsely chopped

   1 cups of Swiss chard

   1 cucumber, rinsed and coarsely chopped

Preparation Method

Run the pears, tomatoes, kale, carrots, celery, apple, cucumber and Swiss chard through a juicer.

Stir to all the juices. Pass through a sieve, if required.

Stir in the orange and lemon juice. Serve!

Pineapple and Pomegranate Cleanser Juice

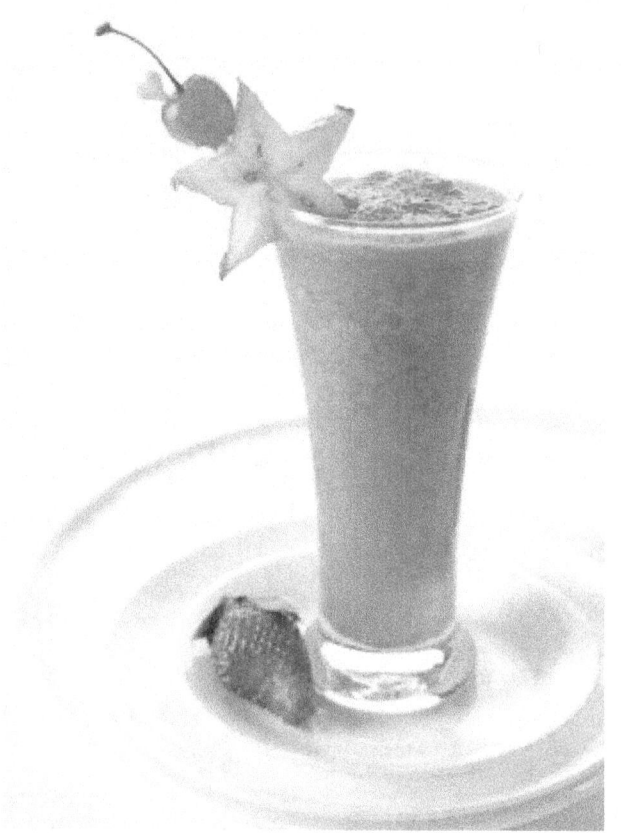

SERVES 3 – 4

Cooking Time: 3 minutes

Nutritional Facts: Calories 69, Protein 0.4 g, Total Fat 0.0 g, Carbohydrates 16.7 g

Ingredients

¾ cup pineapple juice (unsweetened, preferably fresh)

3 cups water

1 lemon, juiced

1 cup pomegranate juice, (unsweetened, preferably fresh)

Preparation Method

Combine all the ingredients and serve.

Tastes best when chilled!

7 – DAY DETOX JUICING PLAN WITH RECIPES

The *7-Day Detox Juicing Plan* consists of 7 juicing recipes, each for a different day of weak. Each of the juice fulfills about one-fourth of the average daily recommended fruits and vegetables (about 5 ½ glasses for a 2,000 calorie diet).

If you are on a pure juicing diet, drink at least 5 glasses of the particular juice per day. Or else you can also follow a nutritional diet and replace your lunch and snack with these juices for 7 days.

Day 1 – Go Green Juice

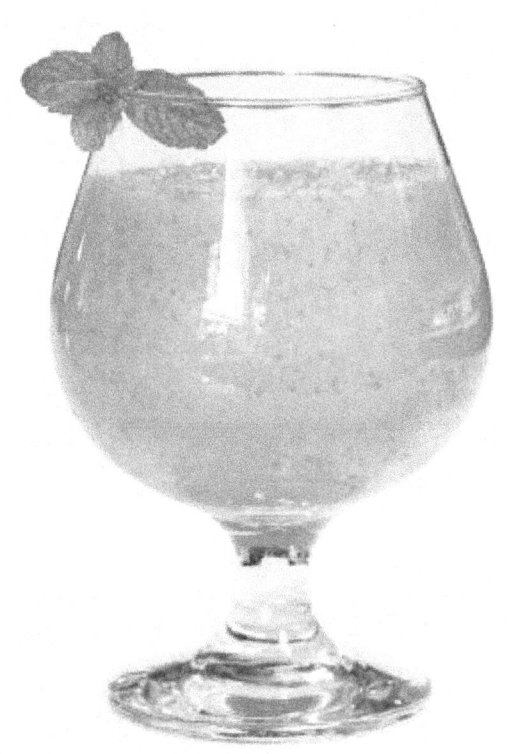

MAKES about 4 cups

Cooking Time: 5 minutes

Nutritional Facts: Calories 91, Protein 1 g, Total Fat 1 g, Carbohydrates 20 g

Ingredients

      2 cups fresh parsley

12 stalks of celery, trimmed

1 lemon, peeled

Ice cubes, as required

6 cups fresh spinach

4 medium pears sized, cut into wedges

Preparation Method

Run all the ingredients through a juicer, in the following sequence:

Parsley – Spinach – Lemon – Pears – Celery

Put 2 – 3 ice cubes in each serving glass.

Pour the juice over the ice cubes.

Drink immediately.

Day 2 – Red Hot Detox Drink

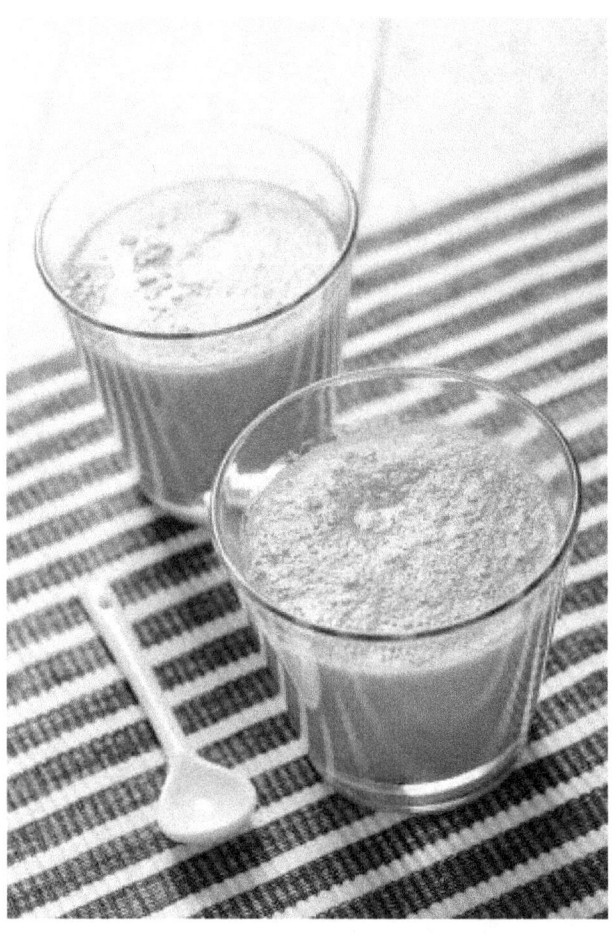

MAKES about 2 cups

Cooking Time: 5 minutes

Nutritional Facts: Calories 46, Protein 1 g, Total Fat 0 g, Carbohydrates 9 g

Ingredients

> 1 cup chopped romaine
>
> 1 red bell pepper, cut into thick strips
>
> 2 large stalks of celery, trimmed
>
> 2 large sized tomatoes, cut into wedges
>
> ¼ cup fresh chives, chopped
>
> 1 medium sized carrot, peeled

¼ fresh jalapeno, remove the stems and seeds

Ice cubes (optional)

Preparation Method

Run all the ingredients through a juicer, in the following sequence:

Romaine – Chives – Tomatoes – Jalapeno – Bell pepper – Celery – Carrot

Put 2 – 3 ice cubes in each serving glass, if using.

Pour the juice over the ice cubes.

Serve immediately.

Day 3 – Cabbage and Berry Juice

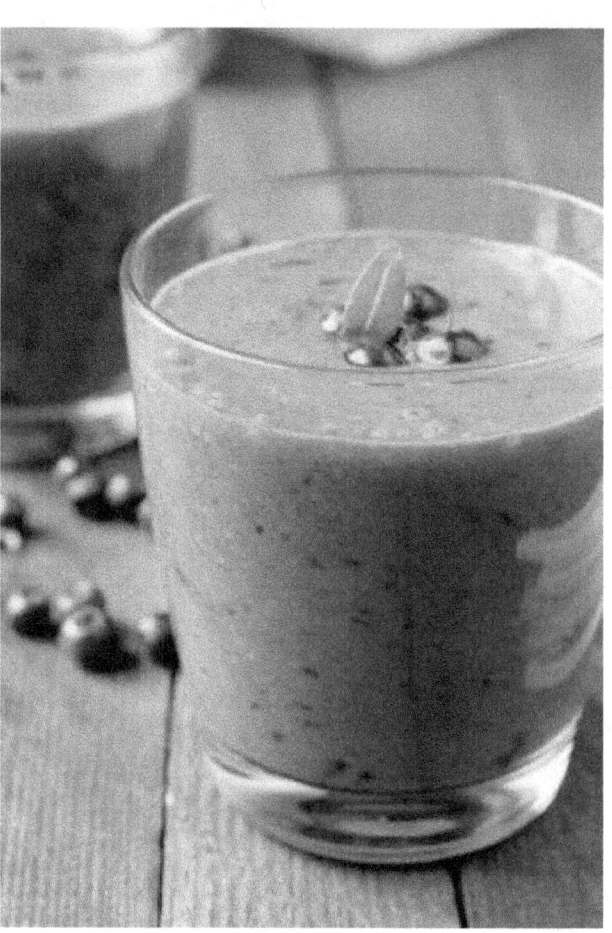

MAKES about 4 cups

Cooking Time: 5 minutes

Nutritional Facts: Calories 77, Protein 1 g, Total Fat 0 g, Carbohydrates 18 g

Ingredients

2 large cucumbers, peeled and cut into thick slices

2 large sized apple, cut into wedges

Half medium sized red cabbage, coarsely sliced

Ice cubes, as required

2 cups fresh blueberries

Preparation Method

Run all the ingredients through a juicer, in the following sequence:

Cabbage – Cucumber – Blueberry – Apples

Put 2 – 3 ice cubes in each serving glass.

Pour the juice over the ice cubes.

Drink immediately.

Day 4 – Sweet Red Juice

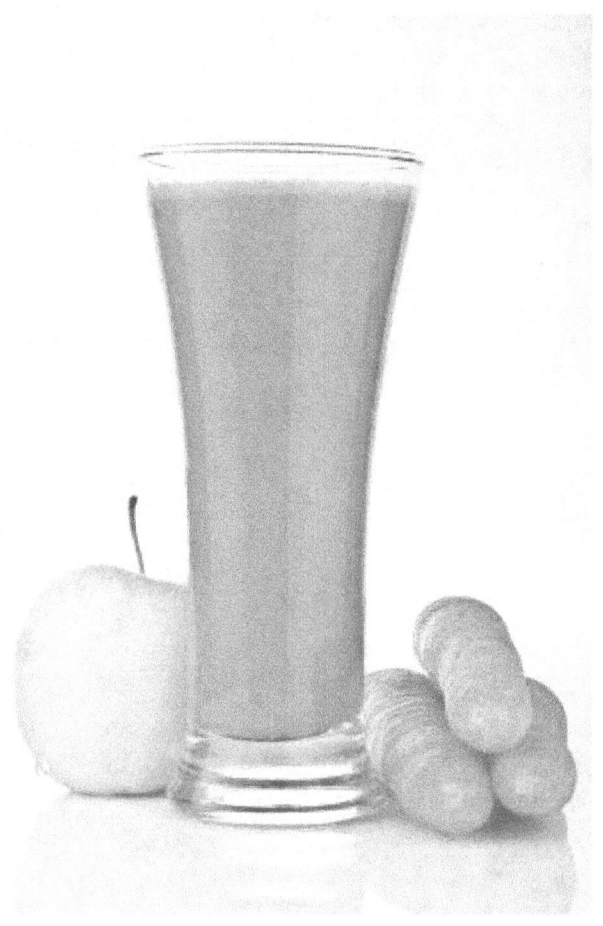

MAKES about 4 cups

Cooking Time: 5 minutes

Nutritional Facts: Calories 69, Protein 1 g, Total Fat 0 g, Carbohydrates 15 g

Ingredients

2 large cucumbers, peeled and thickly sliced

2 medium carrots, peeled

12 fresh strawberries, hulled

Ice cubes

2 large apples, cut into wedges

Preparation Method

Run all the ingredients through a juicer, in the following sequence:

Strawberries – Cucumber – Apple wedges – Carrots

Put 2 – 3 ice cubes in each serving glass.

Pour the juice over the ice cubes.

Serve immediately.

Day 5 – Orange Juicing Reboot

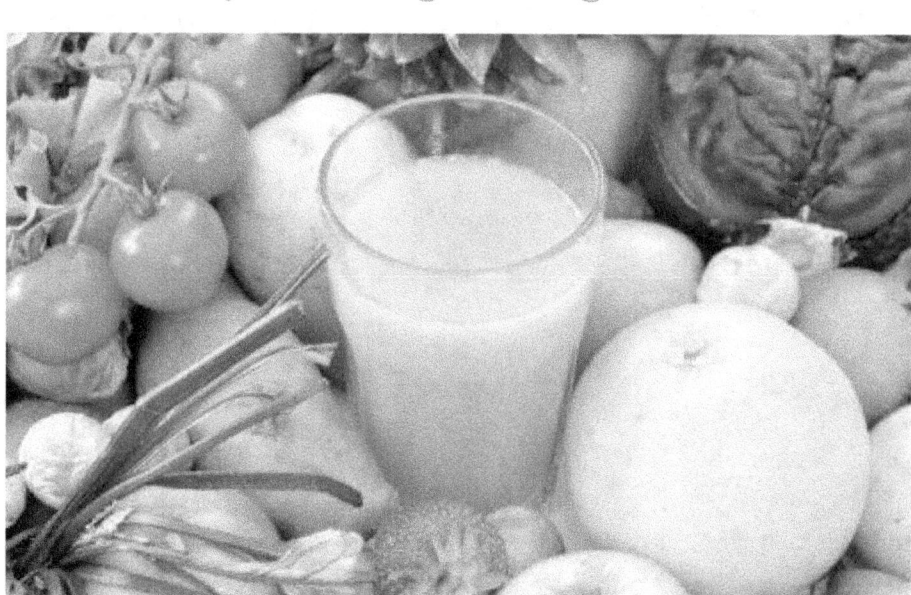

MAKES about 4 cups

Cooking Time: 5 minutes

Nutritional Facts: Calories 111, Protein 2 g, Total Fat 1 g, Carbohydrates 24 g

Ingredients

> 2 oranges, juiced
>
> 8 large carrots, peeled
>
> 2 medium sized yellow tomatoes, cut into wedges
>
> 2 medium sized apples, cut into wedges

Preparation Method

Run the apples, carrots and tomatoes through a juice extractor.

Stir in the orange juice.

Add ice cubes if you want.

Pour it into serving glasses.

Drink immediately.

Day 6 – Spinach and Grapefruit Power Drink

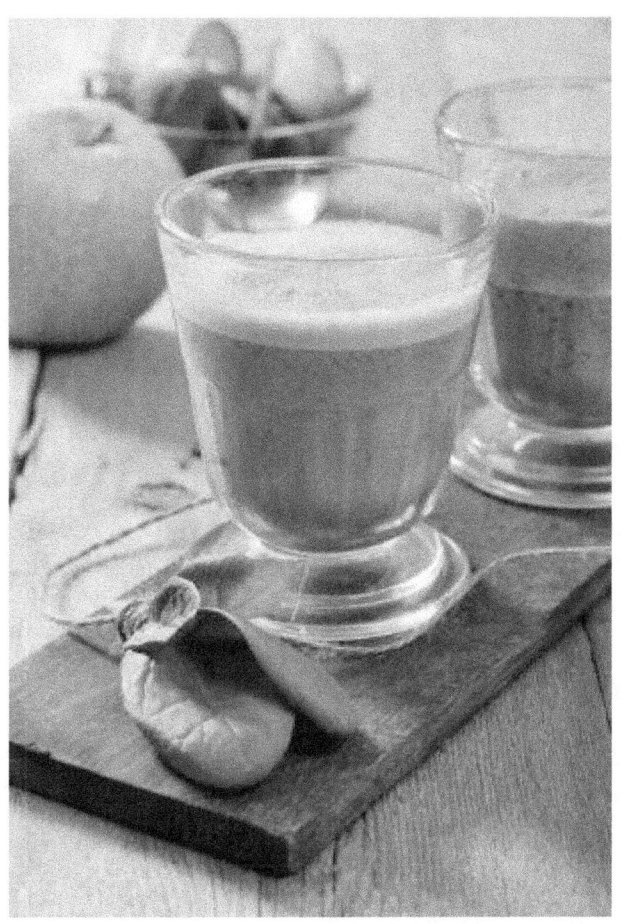

MAKES 4 cups

Cooking Time: 5 minutes

Nutritional Facts: Calories 55, Protein 1 g, Total Fat 0.0 g, Carbohydrates 13 g

Ingredients

>   1 grapefruit, peel and remove the white piths
>
>   1 (2-inch) piece of peeled fresh ginger root
>
>   3 cups fresh spinach
>
>   Ice cubes
>
>   4 large stalks of celery
>
>   4 green apples, cut into wedges

Preparation Method

Run all the ingredients through a juicer, in the following sequence:

Spinach – Grapefruit – Apple wedges – Ginger – Celery

Put 2 – 3 ice cubes in each serving glass.

Pour the juice over the ice cubes.

Serve immediately.

Day 7 – Ginger Orange Juice

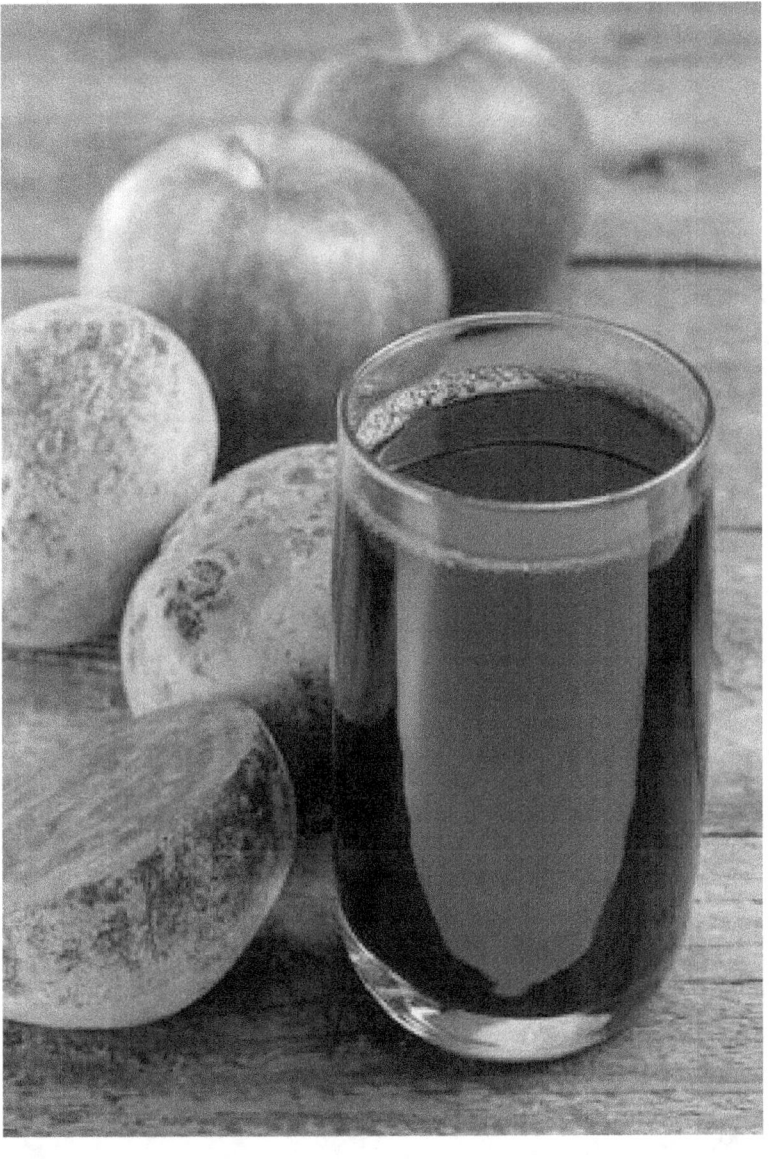

MAKES about 4 cups

Cooking Time: 5 minutes

Nutritional Facts: Calories 100, Protein 2 g, Total Fat 1 g, Carbohydrates 21 g

Ingredients

    2 medium sized oranges, peel and cut into quarters

    2 large beets, peel and cut into wedges

    2 apples, cut into eights

Ice cubes

1 (2-inch) piece of peeled fresh ginger root

6 kale leaves

2 medium carrots, peeled

Preparation Method

Run all the ingredients through a juicer, in the following sequence:

Orange – Kale leaves – Apple– Carrots – Beets – Ginger

Put 2 – 3 ice cubes in each serving glass.

Pour the juice over the ice cubes.

Serve immediately.

5 – DAY JUICING REBOOT WITH RECIPES

The *5 – day juicing reboot* consist of 12 juices, broadly classified into 4 heads; namely Orange drinks, Green drinks, Red drinks and Purple drinks. You need to follow the same plan for 5 consecutive days. There are different recipes under head, so won't get bored of following the same routine.

Following is the daily routine for the *5 – day juicing reboot*.

Early Morning: Drink at least 2 glasses of lukewarm water as soon as you wake up

Breakfast: Drink at least one serving of any orange or red juice (maximum 2 servings)

Mid Morning: Drink 2 cups of coconut water (preferably fresh)

Lunch: Drink one serving of any of the Green Juice

Evening Snack: Drink one serving of any of the Green or Red Juice

Dinner: Drink one serving of any of the Green Juice and one serving of purple or orange juice.

Bedtime: 1 cup of any natural unsweetened herbal tea.

Keep sipping water at frequently regular intervals.

Orange Drinks

Tropical Detox Drink

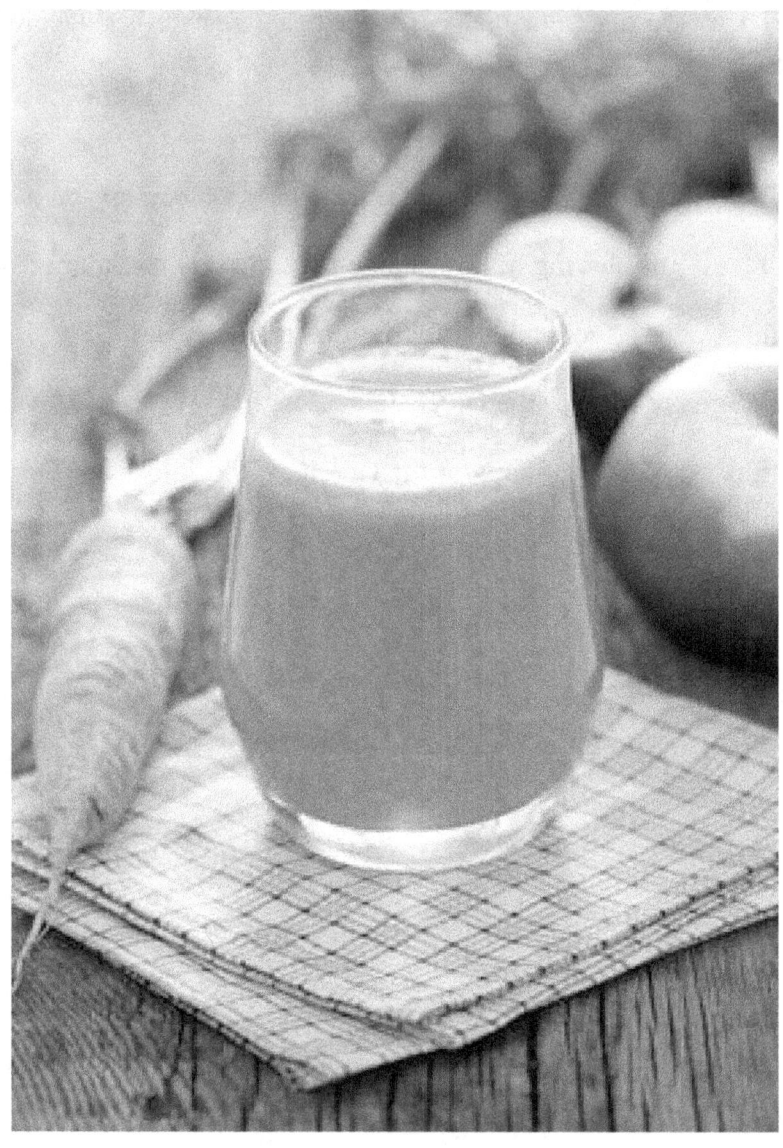

MAKES about 12 ounces of juice (one serving)

Cooking Time: 3 minutes

Nutritional Facts: Calories 274, Protein 4 g, Total Fat 0 g, Carbohydrates 75 g

Ingredients

    4 medium sized carrots, peeled

1 lemon, juiced

2 medium sized apples, cut into wedges

Preparation Method

Run the carrots and apples through an electric juicer.

Stir in the lemon juice.

Drink immediately.

Sweet Ginger Juice

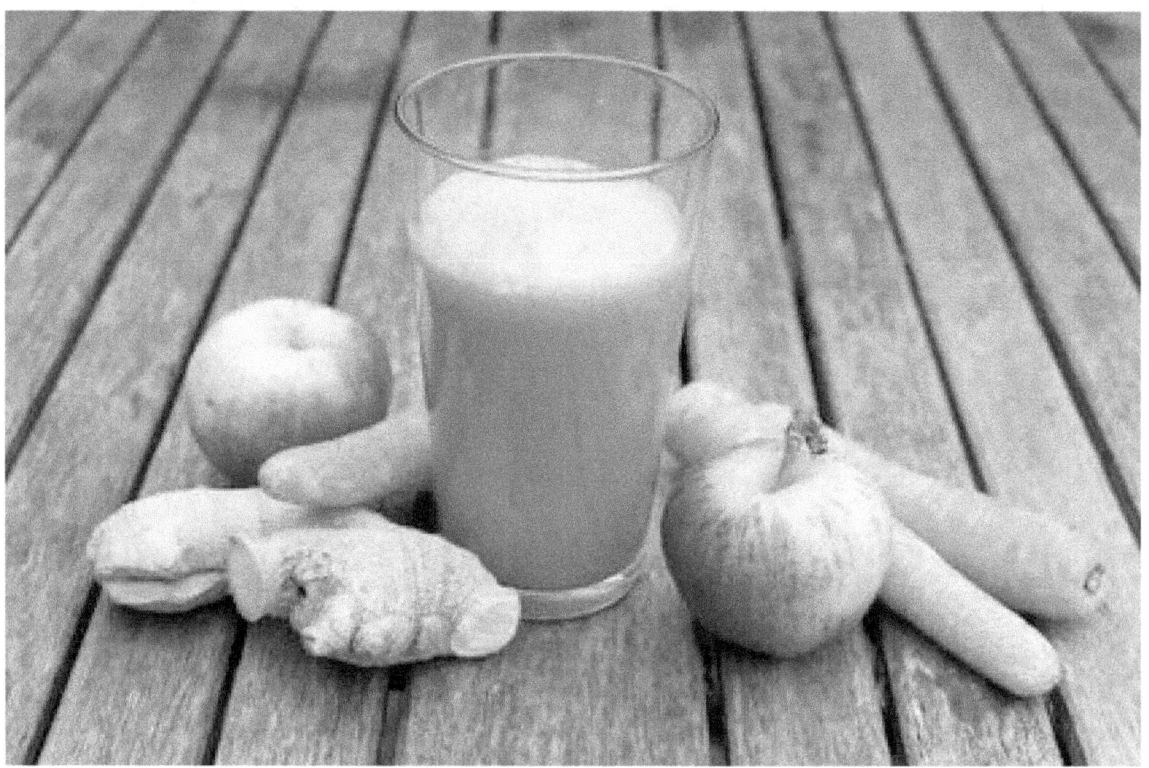

MAKES about 12 ounces of juice (one serving)

Cooking Time: 3 minutes

Nutritional Facts: Calories 265, Protein 3 g, Total Fat 0 g, Carbohydrates 68 g

Ingredients

 2 medium sized apples, cut into wedges

 3 medium sized carrots, peeled

 1 (1-inch) piece of fresh ginger

 Ice cubes (optional)

Preparation Method

Run the carrots, apples and ginger through an electric juicer.

Put 2 – 3 ice cubes in a serving glass.

Pour juice over top of the ice cubes.

Drink immediately.

Sunrise Juicing Reboot

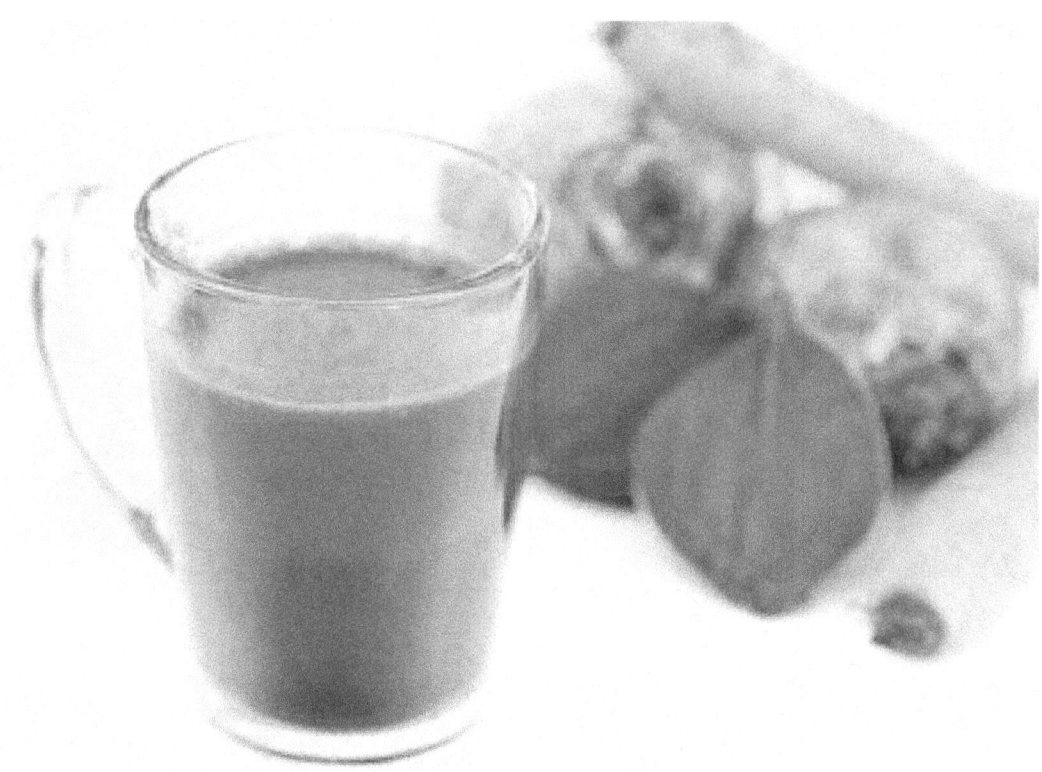

MAKES about 12 ounces of juice (one serving)

Cooking Time: 3 minutes

Nutritional Facts: Calories 191, Protein 5 g, Total Fat 0 g, Carbohydrates 45 g

Ingredients

4 medium sized carrots, peeled

2 oranges, juiced

1 beet, peeled (red cabbage)

Preparation Method

Run the carrots and beets through an electric juicer.

Stir in the orange juice.

Drink immediately.

Green Drinks

Apple and Herbs Drink

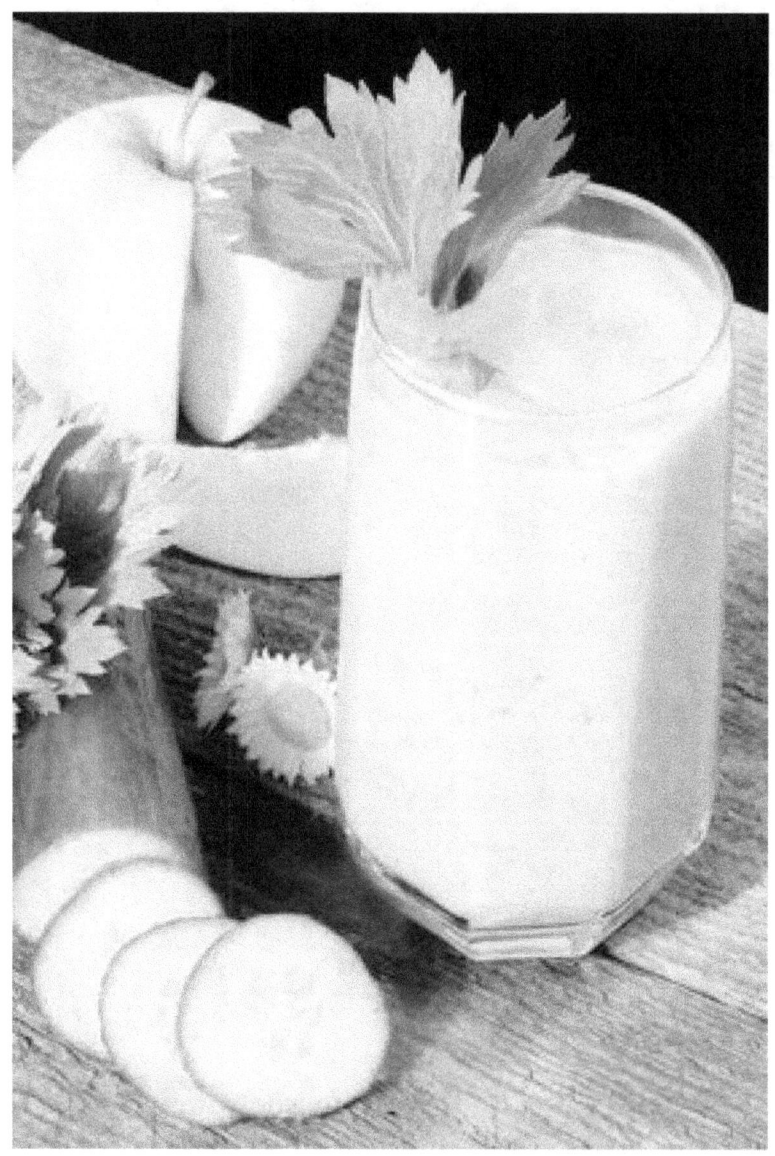

MAKES about 12 ounces of juice (one serving)

Cooking Time: 3 minutes

Nutritional Facts: Calories 284, Protein 4 g, Total Fat 0 g, Carbohydrates 73 g

Ingredients

Handful of parsley

2 green apples, cut into wedges

7 kale leaves

2 cucumbers

Preparation Method

Run all the ingredients through an electric juicer.

Pass the juice through a sieve, if required.

Drink immediately.

Lemon Spiked Green Juice

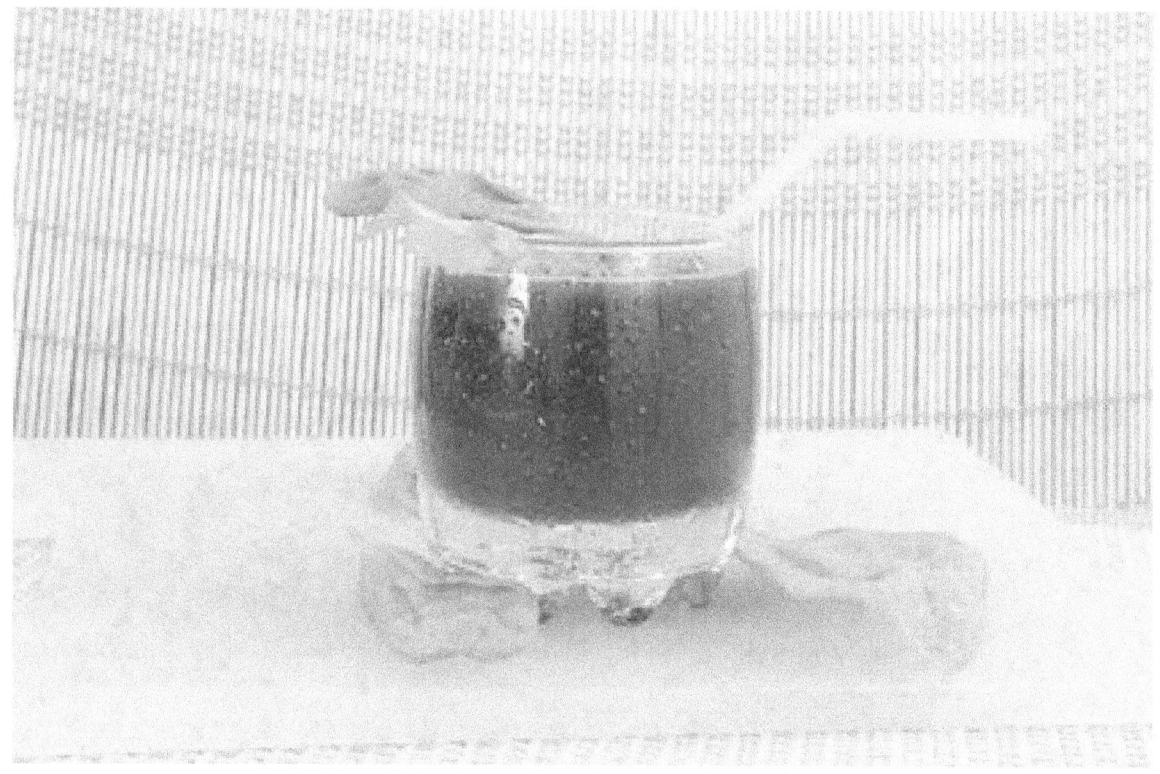

MAKES about 12 ounces of juice (one serving)

Cooking Time: 3 minutes

Nutritional Facts: Calories 163, Protein 5 g, Total Fat 0 g, Carbohydrates 41 g

Ingredients

8 kales leaves

1 cucumber

1 cup fresh spinach

1 lemon, juiced

1 green apple

2 stalks of celery

Preparation Method

Except for lemon juice, run all the other ingredients through an electric juicer.

Pass the juice through a sieve.

Stir in the lemon juice.

Drink immediately.

Kale Lemonade

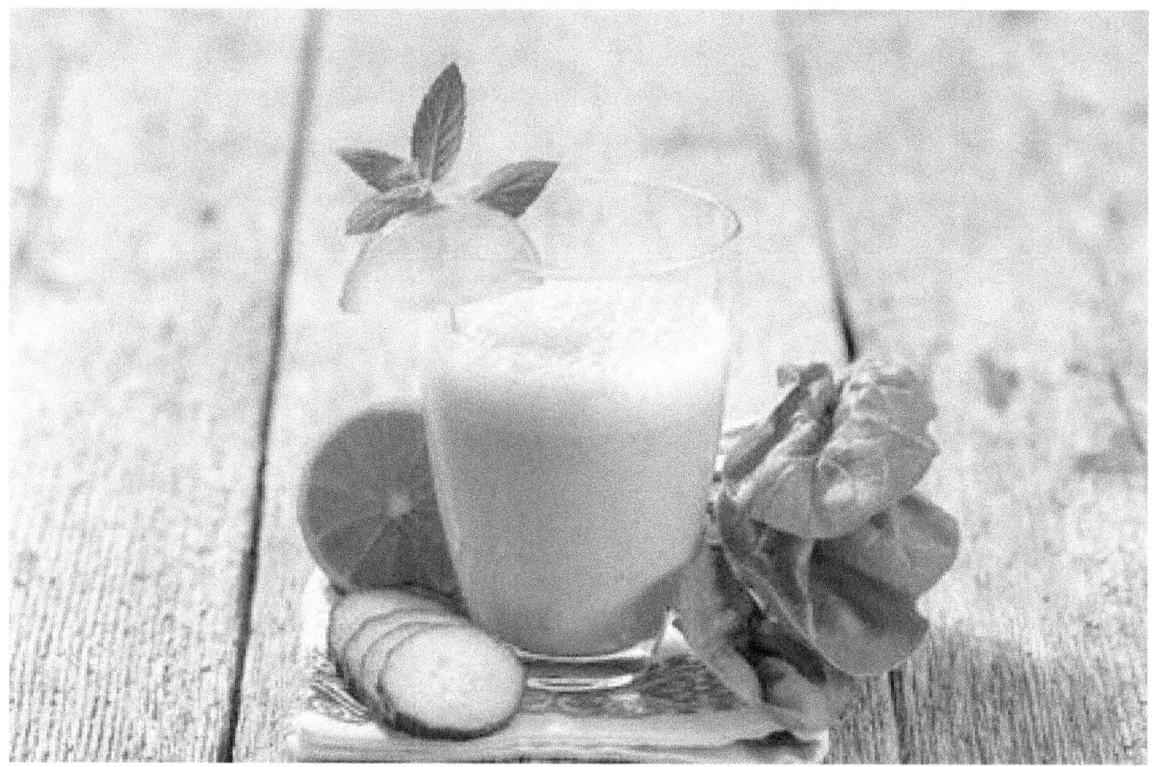

MAKES about 12 ounces of juice (one serving)

Cooking Time: 3 minutes

Nutritional Facts: Calories 154, Protein 4 g, Total Fat 0 g, Carbohydrates 38.5 g

Ingredients

1 medium cucumber

1 green apple, cut into wedges

6 kale leaves

Half lime, juiced

2 celery stalks

1 (1-inch) piece of fresh ginger

Preparation Method

Except for the lime juice, run all the other ingredients through an electric juicer.

Pass the juice through a sieve, if required.

Stir in the lime juice.

Drink immediately.

Red Drinks

Beet-ilicious

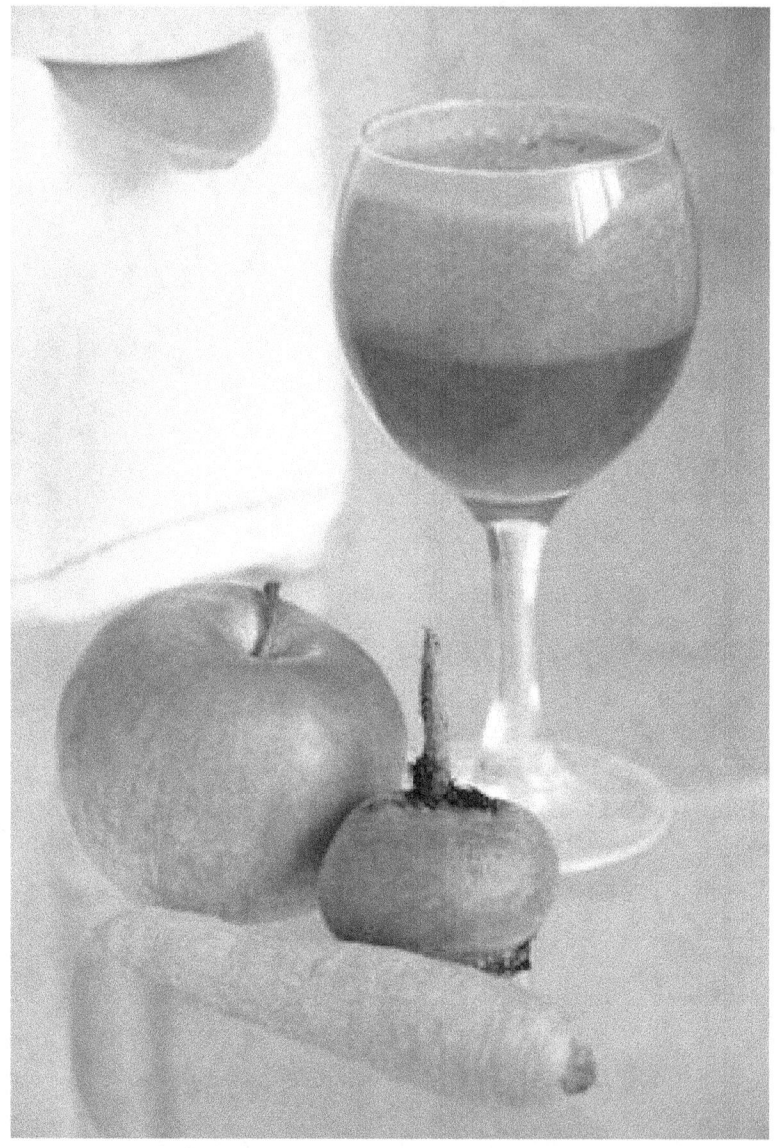

MAKES about 12 ounces of juice (one serving)

Cooking Time: 3 minutes

Nutritional Facts: Calories 205, Protein 3 g, Total Fat 0 g, Carbohydrates 51 g

Ingredients

      1 large red apple, cut into wedges

      1 beet, peeled

1 (1-inch) piece of fresh ginger

3 medium carrots

3 cups kale (substitute: spinach or Swiss chard)

Preparation Method

Run all the ingredients through an electric juicer.

Pass the juice through a sieve, if required.

Drink immediately.

Workout Boost

(Pre/post workout power drink)

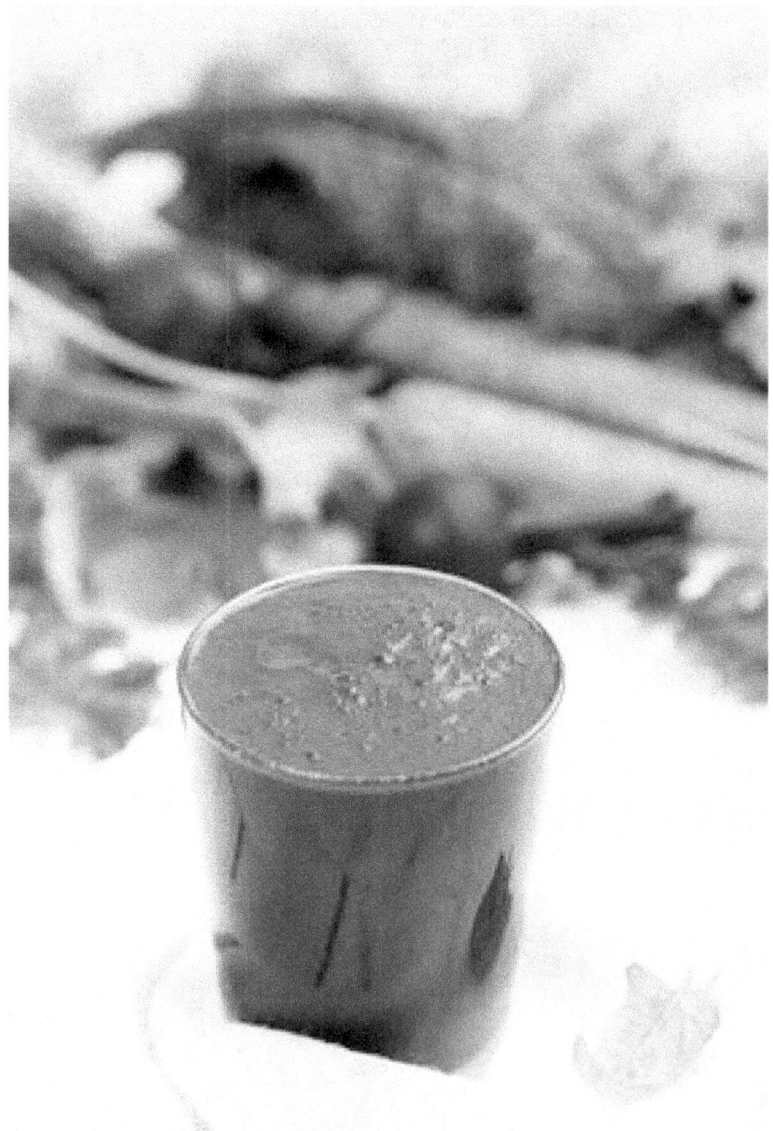

MAKES about 12 ounces of juice (one serving)

Cooking Time: 3 minutes

Nutritional Facts: Calories 145, Protein 1.5 g, Total Fat 0 g, Carbohydrates 33 g

Ingredients

 3 stalks of celery

 1 medium carrot, peeled

Half lemon

Handful of basil leaves

2 beets, peeled

1 orange, peeled and halved

Preparation Method

Except for the lemon, run all the other ingredients through an electric juicer.

Pass the juice through a sieve, if required.

Squeeze in the lemon. Stir to mix.

Drink immediately.

Watermelon Lovers

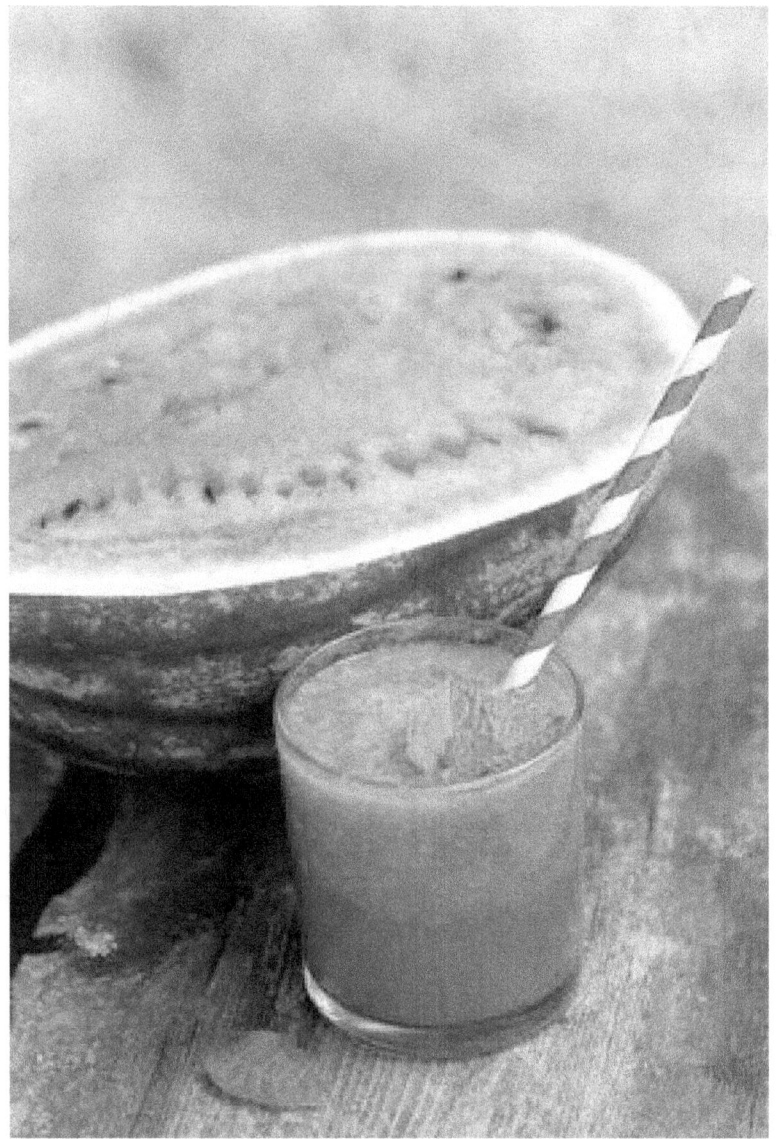

MAKES about 12 ounces of juice (one serving)

Cooking Time: 3 minutes

Nutritional Facts: Calories 140, Protein 2.6 g, Total Fat 0 g, Carbohydrates 33.5 g

Ingredients

Half medium sized watermelon, cut the meat to fit in the juicers size

Handful of basil

1 lime, juiced

Ice cubes

Preparation Method

Run the basil and watermelon through an electric juicer.

Stir in the lime juice.

Put ice cubes in it.

Drink immediately.

Fruity Sweet Potato Surprise

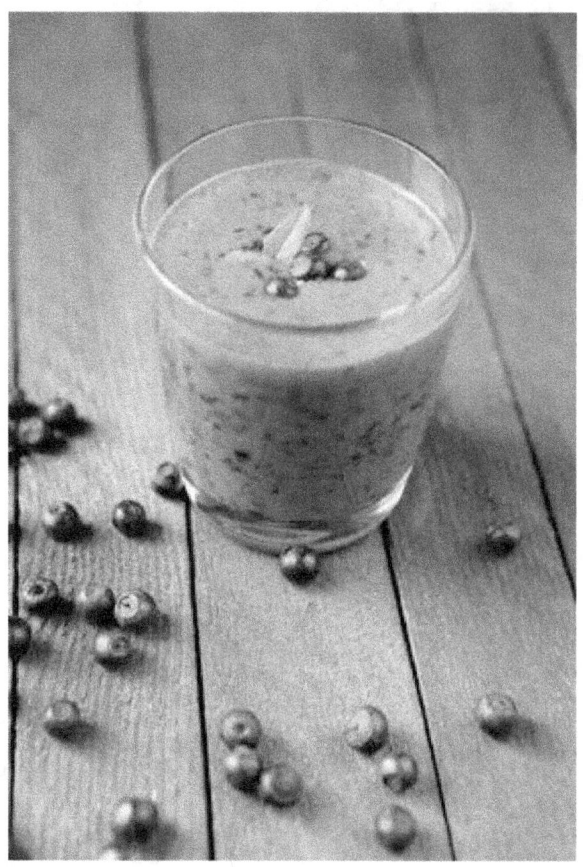

MAKES about 12 ounces of juice (one serving)

Cooking Time: 3 minutes

Nutritional Facts: Calories 296, Protein 3.5 g, Total Fat 0.5 g, Carbohydrates 73.5 g

Ingredients

    1 sweet potato, washed and peeled

    Handful of fresh blueberries

    2 ripe peaches, pitted (substitute: ripe pears)

    Pinch of ground cinnamon

    1 red apple, cut into wedges

Preparation Method

Juice the sweet potato, blueberries, apples and peaches. Stir to mix.

Stir in the cinnamon.

Drink immediately.

Purple Grapes Delight

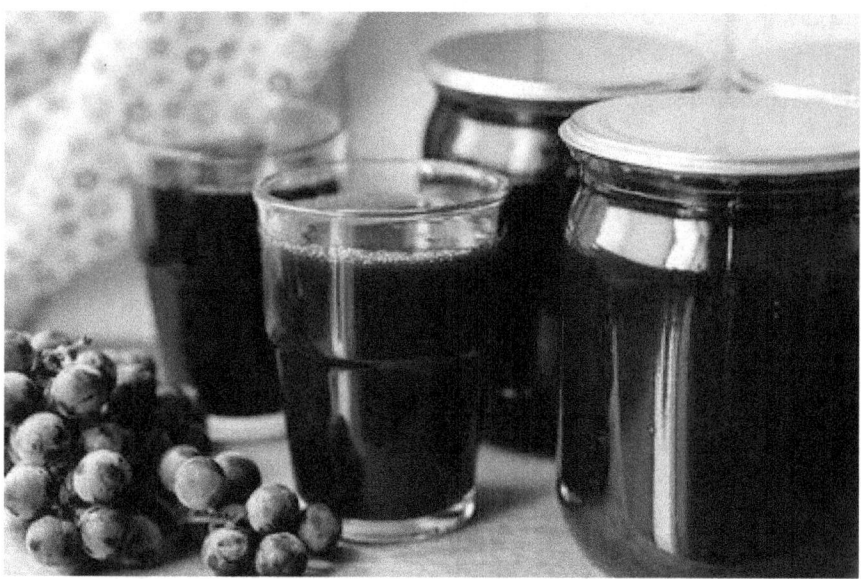

MAKES about 12 ounces of juice (one serving)

Cooking Time: 3 minutes

Nutritional Facts: Calories 224, Protein 3 g, Total Fat 2 g, Carbohydrates 71 g

Ingredients

> 2 cups fresh blueberries
>
> 30 black or red grapes
>
> Handful of fresh mint leaves
>
> 2 – 3 ice cubes

Preparation Method

Run all the ingredients through an electric juicer.

Pass the juice through a sieve, if required.

Add ice cubes.

Drink immediately.

Blue Kale Drink

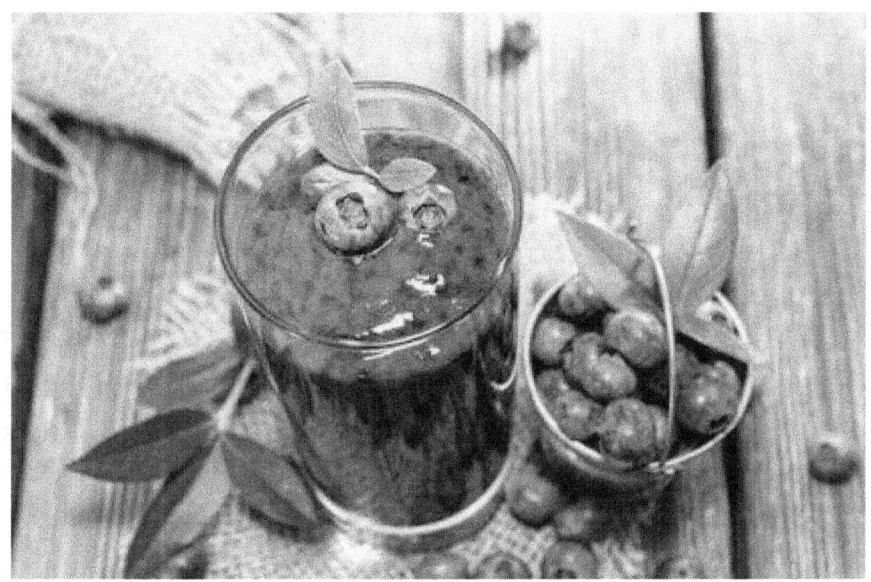

MAKES about 12 ounces of juice (one serving)

Cooking Time: 3 minutes

Nutritional Facts: Calories 96, Protein 2 g, Total Fat 1 g, Carbohydrates 25 g

Ingredients

> 1 cup blueberries
>
> ¼ watermelon, cut the meat of the watermelon to fit in the juicers size
>
> 7 kale leaves

Preparation Method

Juice all the ingredients. Stir to mix.

Pass the juice through a sieve, if required.

Drink immediately.

Spinach Berry Riser

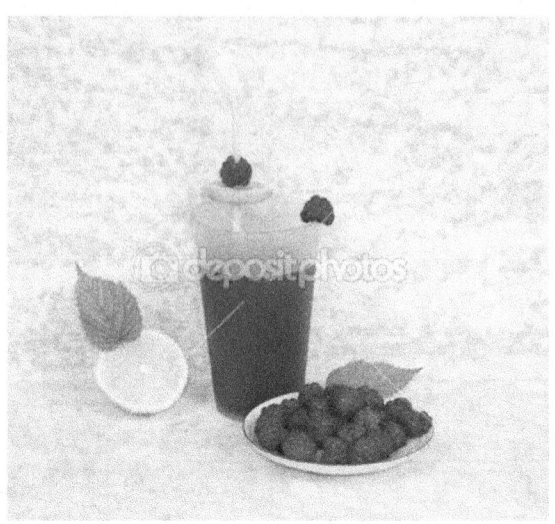

SERVES 1

Cooking Time: 3 minutes

Nutritional Facts: Calories 318, Protein 6.5 g, Total Fat 12 g, Carbohydrates 49 g

Ingredients

> 1 cup water
>
> ¼ cup fresh spinach
>
> 1 Tbsp flax seed
>
> 1 medium banana
>
> 1 cup fresh raspberries
>
> 1 Tbsp almond butter
>
> 1 tsp fresh lemon juice

Preparation Method

Except for lemon juice, combine all the other ingredients in a food processor.

Pulse till it becomes a smoothie.

Stir in the lemon juice.

Enjoy!

Green Almond Smoothie

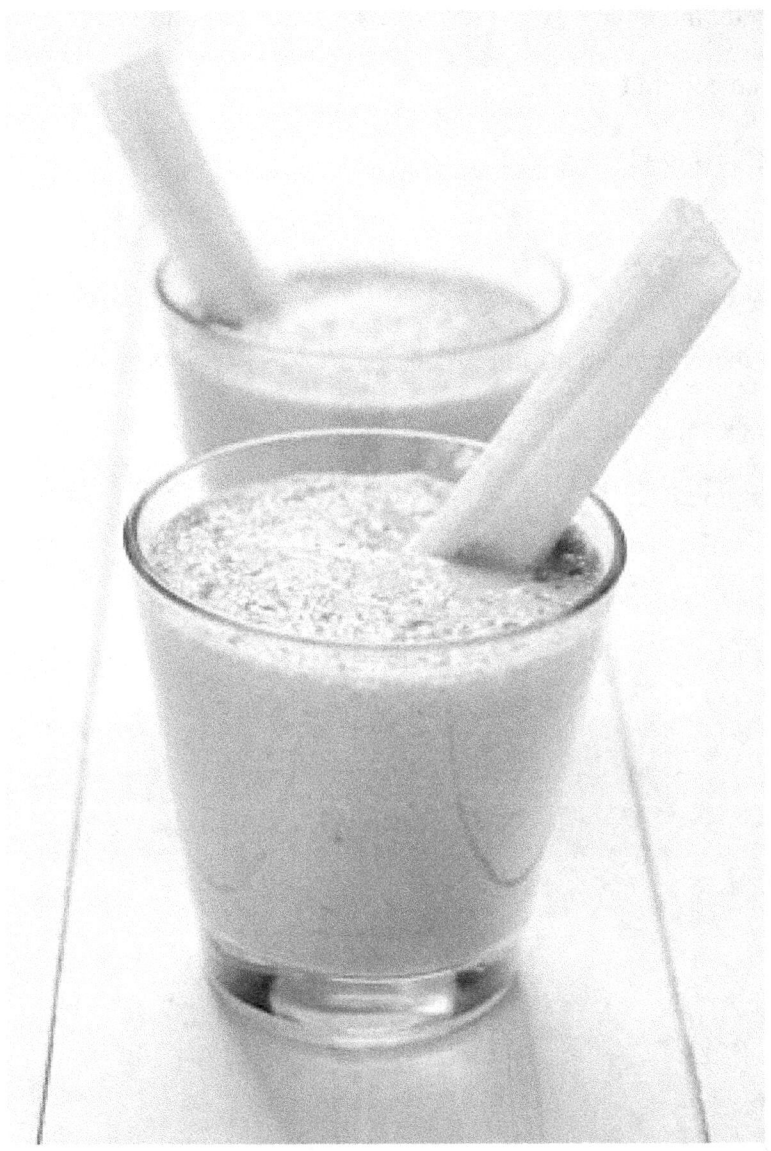

SERVES 1

Cooking Time: 3 minutes

Nutritional Facts: Calories 375, Protein 5.5 g, Total Fat 15.5 g, Carbohydrates 60 g

Ingredients

Half cup almond milk

4 stalks of celery

1 cup kale

1 medium cucumber

1 cup chopped pineapple

1 Tbsp melted coconut oil

Half green apple, juiced

Half lime, juiced

Preparation Method

Combine the first 6 ingredients in a food processor.

Blend till it becomes a smoothie.

Stir in the apple and lime juice.

Drink immediately.

Fruity Avocado Coconut Water

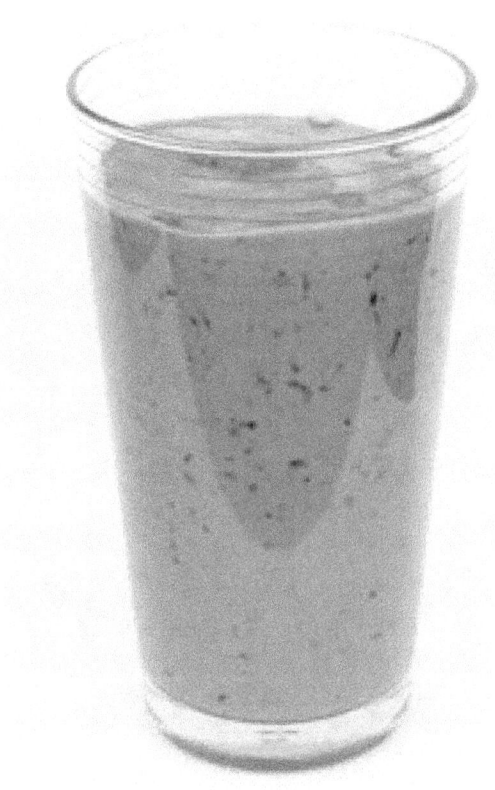

SERVES 2

Cooking Time: 3 minutes

Nutritional Facts: Calories 304, Protein 4.5 g, Total Fat 16.5 g, Carbohydrates 36.5 g

Ingredients

½ cup diced mango

1½ cup coconut water

1 cup kale

½ tsp cayenne pepper

1 cup blueberries

1 Tbsp fresh lemon juice

1 small ripe avocado

1 Tbsp flaxseed

Preparation Method

Except for lemon juice, combine all the other ingredients in a food processor.

Pulse till it becomes a smoothie.

Stir in the lemon juice.

Drink immediately.

LIVER DETOX DRINKS

Grapefruit Delight

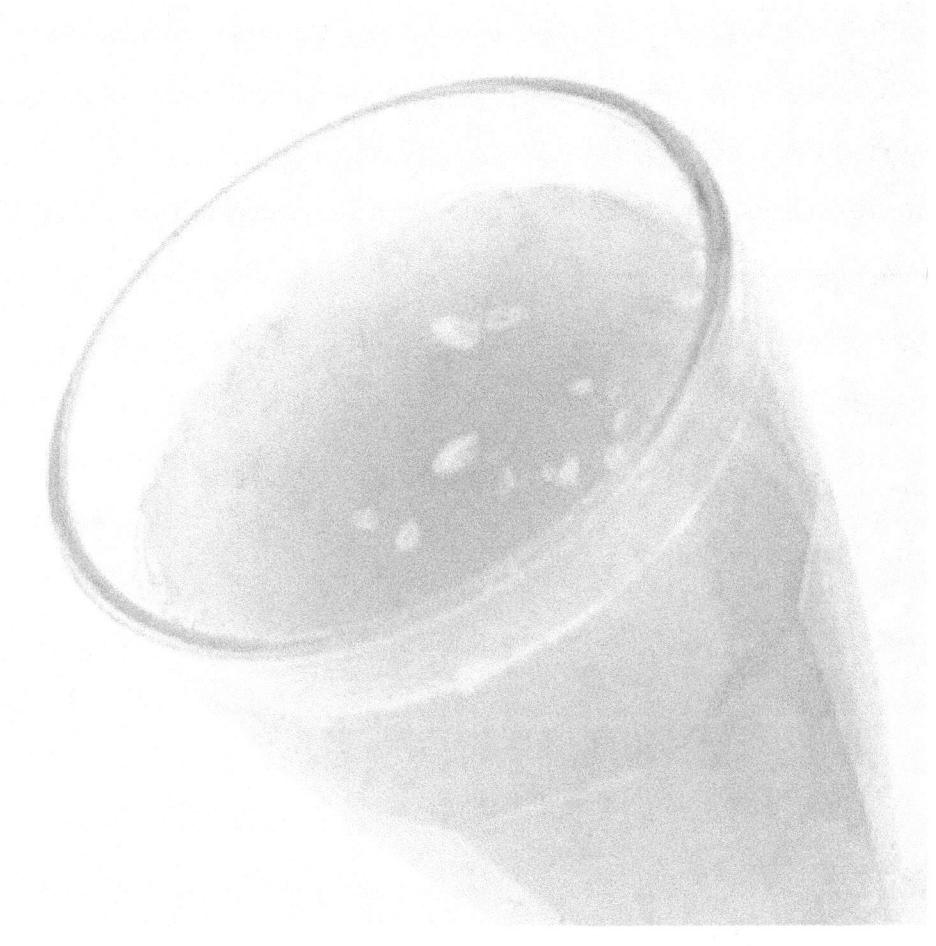

SERVES 1

Cooking Time: 3 minutes

Nutritional Facts: Calories 316, Protein 4 g, Total Fat 3 g, Carbohydrates 72

Ingredients

500 ml water (about 2 ¼ cups), boiled and cooled

3 Tbsp flaxseed oil

1 (4-inch) piece of fresh ginger root

½ tsp ground cumin powder

4 cloves of garlic, peeled

6 lemons, juiced

4 leaves of fresh Mint

3 grapefruits, juiced

Preparation Method

Combine the water, garlic and ginger in a food processor.

Pulse till thoroughly blended. Transfer it to a glass through a sieve. Discard the residues.

Stir in the lemon and grapefruit juice.

Return it to the processor along with the flaxseed oil and cumin.

Pulse for 45 seconds.

Pour it in a serving glass.

Garnish with mint leaves and enjoy!

Pear and Celery Detoxifier

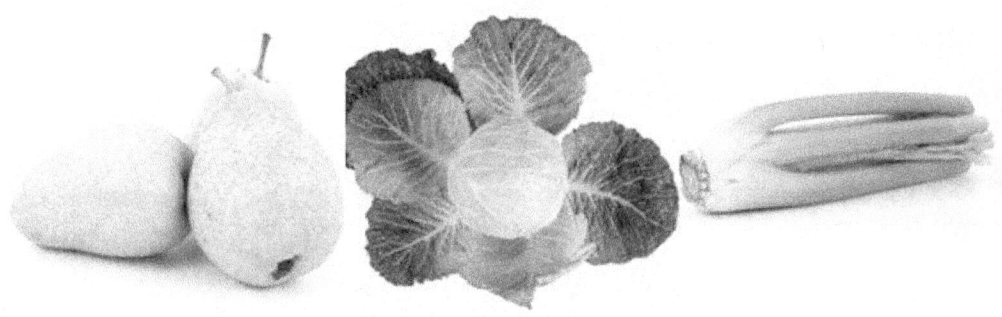

SERVES 1

Cooking Time: 2 minutes

Nutritional Facts: Calories 156, Protein 1.2 g, Total Fat 0.3 g, Carbohydrates 40 g

Ingredients

> 1 large lemon, juiced
>
> 250 grams fresh pears, chopped
>
> 12g grams fresh cabbage, chopped
>
> 1 (1-inch) slice of fresh ginger root, chopped
>
> 25 grams celery, chopped
>
> 500 ml filtered Water (about 2 ¼ cups)

Preparation Method

Except for the lemon juice, combine all the other ingredients in a food processor.

Pulse for 1 minute.

Stir in the lemon juice.

Serve chilled!

Citrus and Ginger Liver Detox Drink

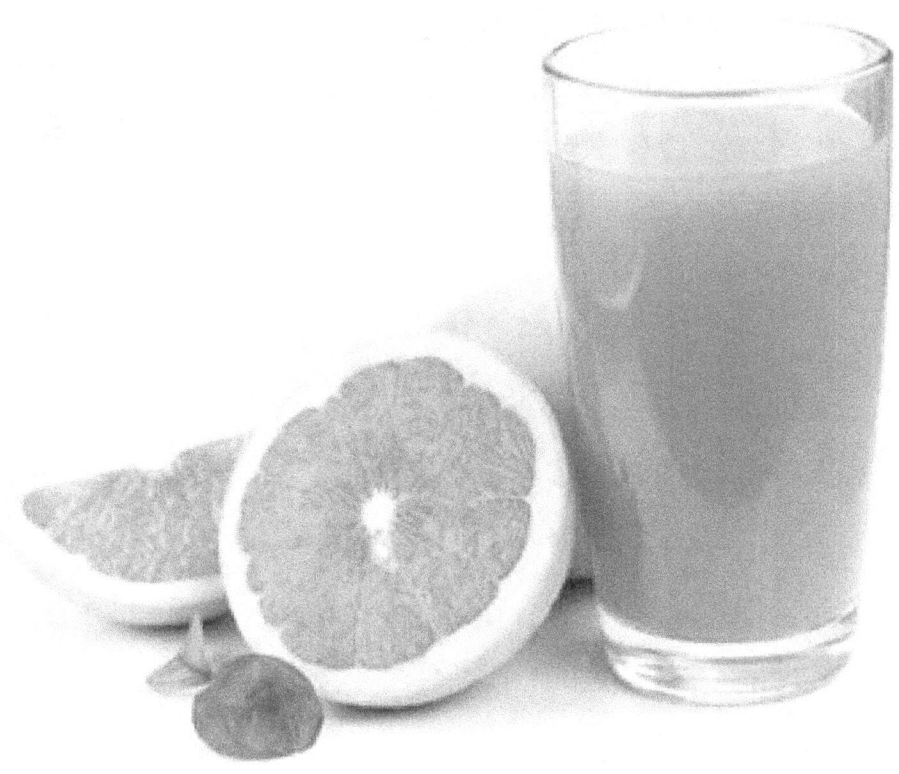

SERVES 1

Cooking Time: 3 minutes

Nutritional Facts: Calories 426, Protein 2 g, Total Fat 28 g, Carbohydrates 44 g

Ingredients

      300 ml distilled water (about 1 ¼ cup)

      1 (2-inch) slice of fresh ginger root, grated

      2 cloves of garlic, peeled and grated

      2 Tbsp cold pressed flax oil

      2 large grapefruits, juiced

      Pinch of cayenne pepper

      4 lemons, juiced

Preparation Method

Extract the juice of ginger and garlic, and put it in a food processor along with all the other ingredients.

Pulse for 45 seconds.

Drink immediately.

Lemon Ginger Detox Drink

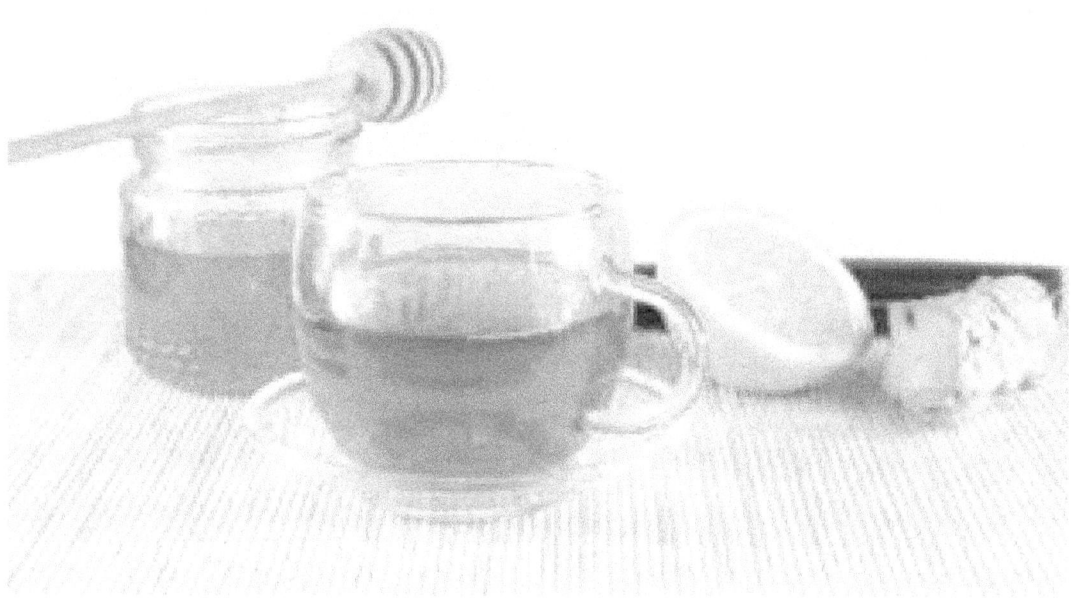

SERVES 2

Cooking Time: 2 minutes

Nutritional Facts: Calories 77, Protein 0.3 g, Total Fat 0.2 g, Carbohydrates 20.7 g

Ingredients

> 1 cup fresh lemon juice
>
> 1 tsp ground ginger
>
> 2 Tbsp honey
>
> 1 tsp ground turmeric
>
> 2 cups distilled water

Preparation Method

Take 2 serving glasses and fill each with 1 cup of distilled water.

Divide all the other ingredients equally between the two glasses.

Stir and serve!

Apple Cider Detox Water

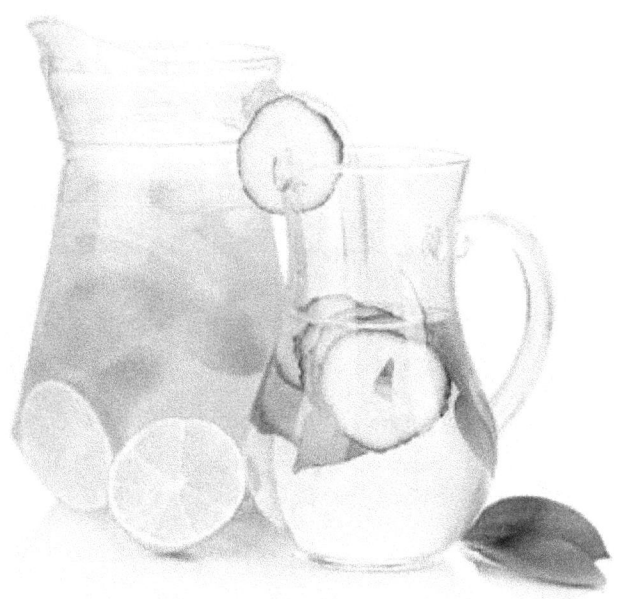

MAKES 2 quarts (Drink throughout the day)

Cooking Time: 3 minutes (overnight refrigeration)

Nutritional Facts: Calories 54, Protein 2 g, Total Fat 0 g, Carbohydrates 12 g

Ingredients

> 1 small cucumber, cut into thin slices
>
> 2 quarts filtered water (about 8 cups)
>
> 1 lemon, cut into thin slices
>
> 6 Tbsp apple cider vinegar
>
> 4 sprigs of mint

Preparation Method

Combine all the ingredients in a bottle or pitcher.

Refrigerate overnight.

Drink it throughout the day, after regular intervals.

JUICING REBOOT RECIPES

Radish Fruit Juicing Reboot

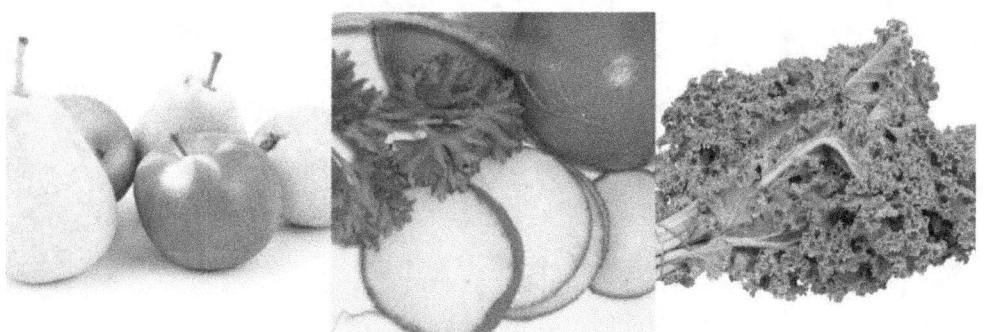

SERVES 2

Cooking Time: 3 minutes

Nutritional Facts: Calories 250, Protein 3.7 g, Total Fat 0.0 g, Carbohydrates 64 g

Ingredients

2 small apples, cored and cut into wedges

1/2 fennel bulb, cut in half

2 large radishes, ends trimmed and coarsely chopped to fit in the juicer

4 kale leaves

2 pears, cored and cut into wedges

Preparation Method

Juice all the ingredients. Stir to mix.

Pass the juice through a sieve, if required.

Drink immediately.

Radish and Jicama Juice

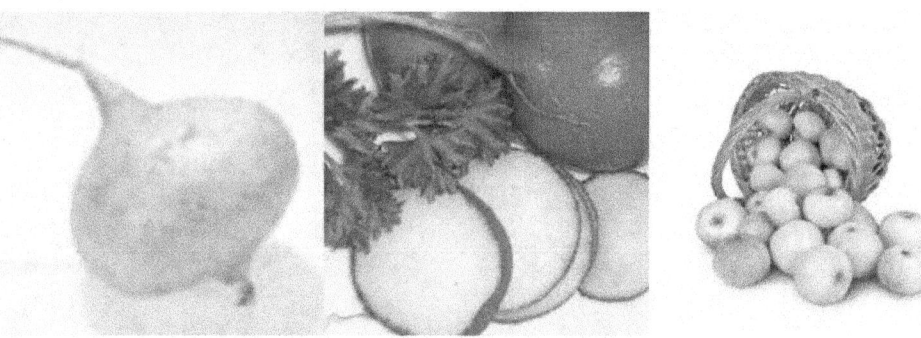

SERVES 2

Cooking Time: 3 minutes

Nutritional Facts: Calories 222, Protein 2.5 g, Total Fat 0.5 g, Carbohydrates 54.5 g

Ingredients

2 large radishes, ends trimmed and coarsely chopped to fit in the juicer

Half cup fresh cilantro

1 jicama

Pinch of sea salt

2 apples, cored and cut into wedges

1 lime, juiced

Preparation Method

Except for the lemon juice, pass all the other ingredients through a juicer. Stir to mix.

Pass the juice through a sieve, if required.

Stir in the lemon juice.

Drink immediately.

Sweet Potato and Orange Drink

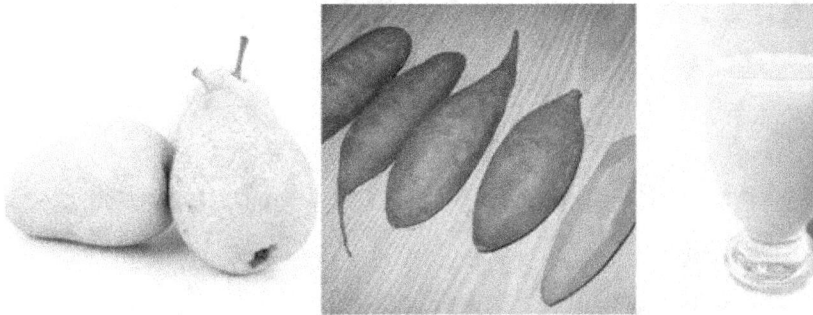

SERVES 2

Cooking Time: 3 minutes

Nutritional Facts: Calories 299, Protein 6.5 g, Total Fat 0.0 g, Carbohydrates 72.5 g

Ingredients

 8 green lettuce leaves

 2 zucchinis

 2 sweet potatoes, peeled

 2 oranges, peeled

 2 pears, cored and cut into wedges

 2 handfuls of dandelion greens

Preparation Method

Juice all the ingredients. Stir to mix.

Pass the juice through a sieve, if required.

Enjoy!

Green Rhubarb Juice

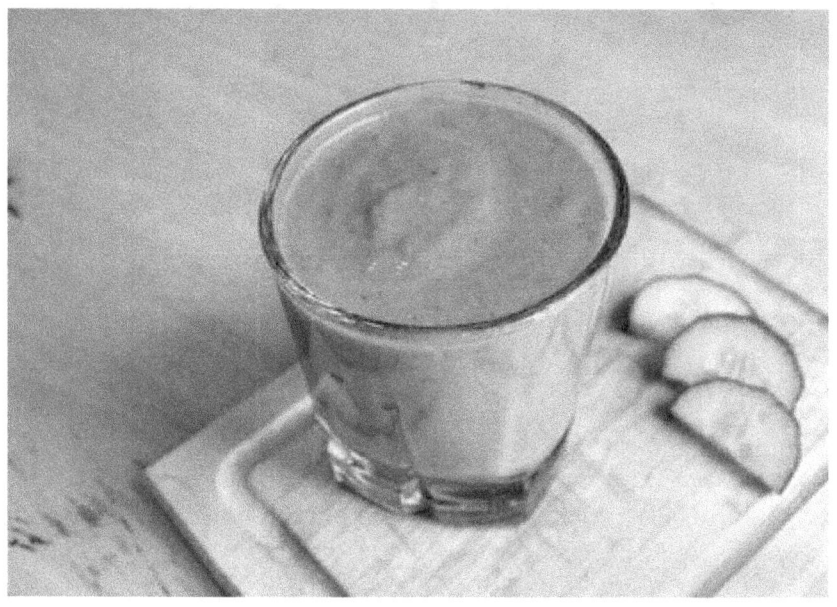

SERVES 2

Cooking Time: 3 minutes

Nutritional Facts: Calories 185, Protein 4 g, Total Fat 0.1 g, Carbohydrates 45 g

Ingredients

12 kale leaves

2 rhubarb stalks, leaves removed

2 apples, cored and cut into wedges

1 (2-inch) piece of fresh ginger root

2 cucumbers, coarsely chopped to fit in the juicer

Preparation Method

Juice all the ingredients. Stir to mix.

Pass the juice through a sieve, if required. Discard the residues.

Enjoy!

Green and Bean juice

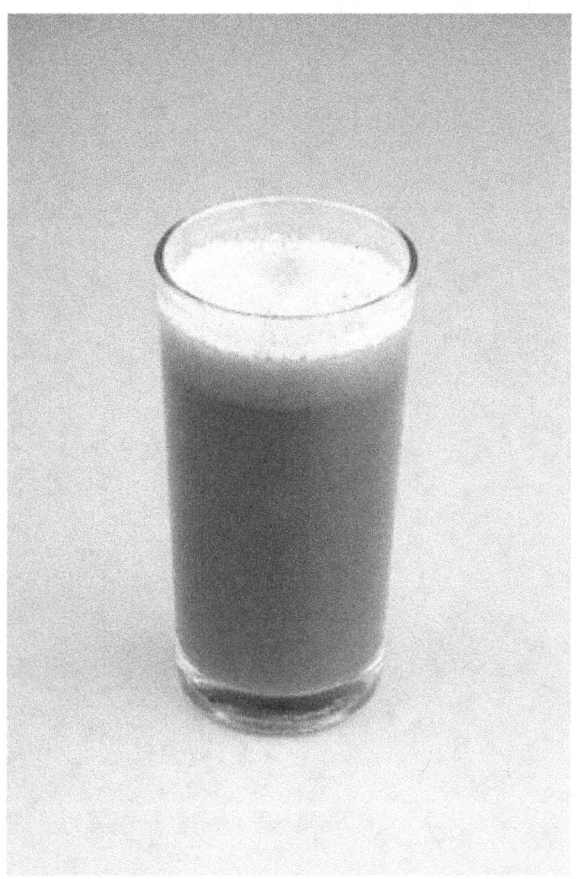

SERVES 2

Cooking Time: 3 minutes

Nutritional Facts: Calories 204, Protein 13 g, Total Fat 1.4 g, Carbohydrates 44.5 g

Ingredients

4 cucumbers, coarsely diced

400 grams green beans

2 lemons, juiced

400 grams spinach

Preparation Method

Except for the lemon juice, pass all the other ingredients through a juicer. Stir to mix.

Pass the juice through a sieve. Discard the residues.

Stir in the lemon juice.

Enjoy!

Spicy Butternut Juice

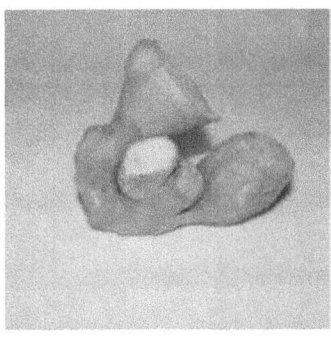 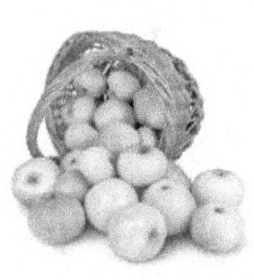 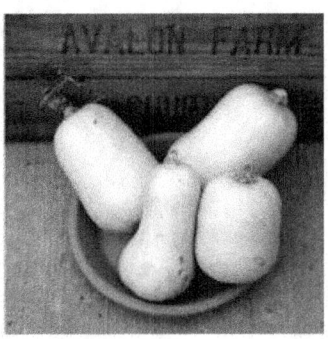

SERVES 2

Cooking Time: 3 minutes

Nutritional Facts: Calories 384, Protein 6 g, Total Fat 0.2 g, Carbohydrates 98 g

Ingredients

> 2 butternut squash, peeled and coarsely chopped
>
> 2 Tbsp apple pie spice mix (substitute: ground cinnamon)
>
> 2 tsp honey
>
> 1 (2-inch) piece of fresh ginger root
>
> 4 apples, cored and cut into wedges
>
> 2 tsp coconut sugar

Preparation Method

Combine coconut sugar and spice in a bowl. Set aside.

Juice the apples, ginger and squash.

Stir in the honey.

Sprinkle the spice-sugar mixture and serve!

Tropical Watermelon Delight .

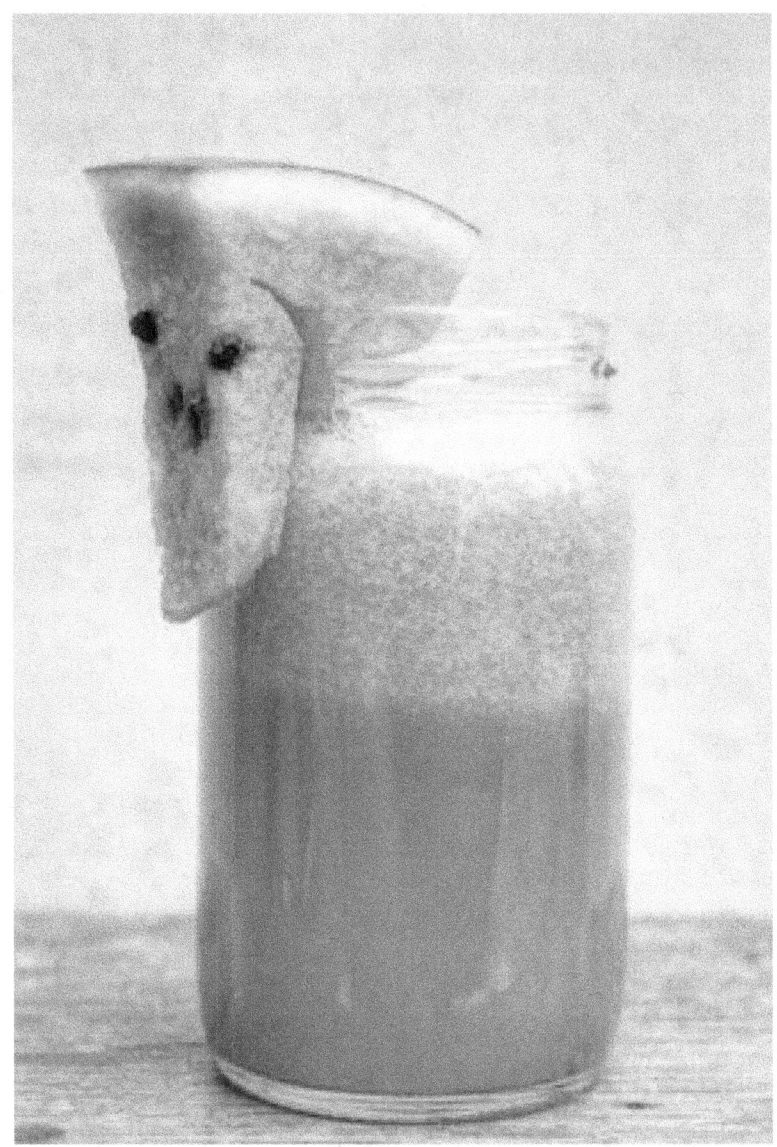

SERVES 2

Cooking Time: 5 minutes

Nutritional Facts: Calories 87.5, Protein 2.5 g, Total Fat 0.0 g, Carbohydrates 21 g

Ingredients

    1 small watermelon

    1 fennel bulb

    1 red cabbage, cut into quarters

2 oranges, peeled and juiced

Preparation Method

Combine the watermelon and cabbage in a food processor.

Pulse till thoroughly blended.

Pass it through a sieve. Discard the residues.

Juice the fennel bulb.

Stir it in the watermelon-cabbage juice.

Finally, stir in the orange juice.

Serve chilled!

Exotic Sweet Potato Smoothie

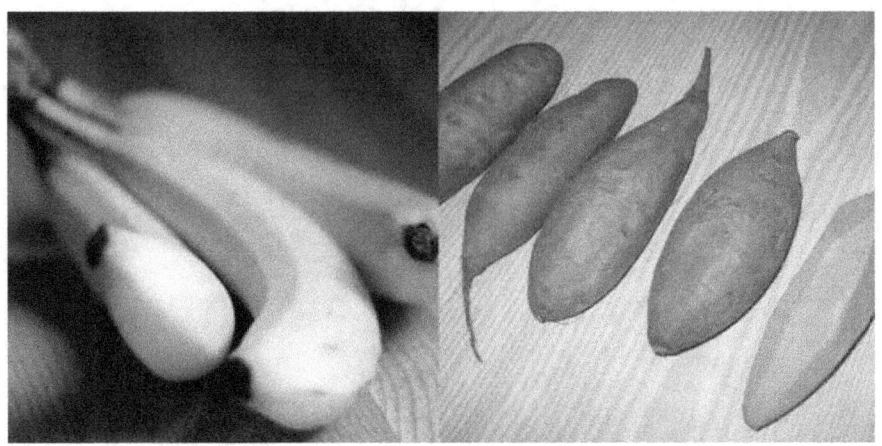

SERVES 2

Cooking Time: 2 minutes

Nutritional Facts: Calories 290, Protein 9 g, Total Fat 14 g, Carbohydrates 37 g

Ingredients

    2 Tbsp almond butter

    500 ml almond milk (about 2 cups)

    ½ tsp ground cinnamon

    1 cup mashed sweet potato

    2 Tbsp ground flax meal

    2 Tbsp coconut oil

    1 medium banana

    1 cup pulp of any green leaf (kale or spinach)

    Pinch of ground cardamom

Preparation Method

Combine all the ingredients in a processor.

Blend till it becomes a smoothie.

Enjoy!

Green Honeydew Smoothie

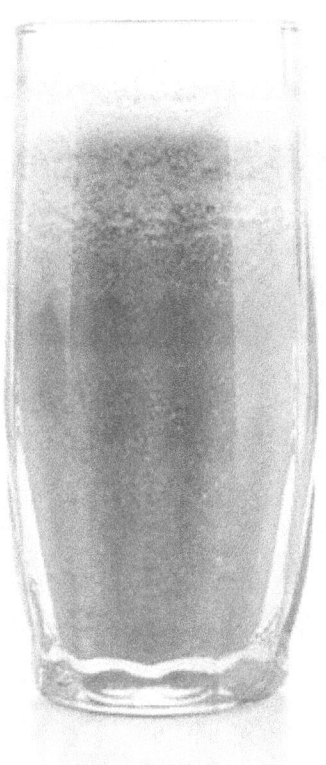

SERVES 2

Cooking Time: 3 minutes

Nutritional Facts: Calories 150, Protein 3 g, Total Fat 0 g, Carbohydrates 35 g

Ingredients

> 500 ml coconut water
>
> 400 grams spinach
>
> 4 – 6 ice cubes
>
> 400 grams honeydew

Preparation Method

Remove the rind and seeds of the honeydew. Peel off its skin and chop coarsely.

Put the chopped honeydew in the food processor along with the spinach and coconut water.

Pulse till thoroughly blended.

Pour it over ice and serve!

Pomegranate Coconut Water

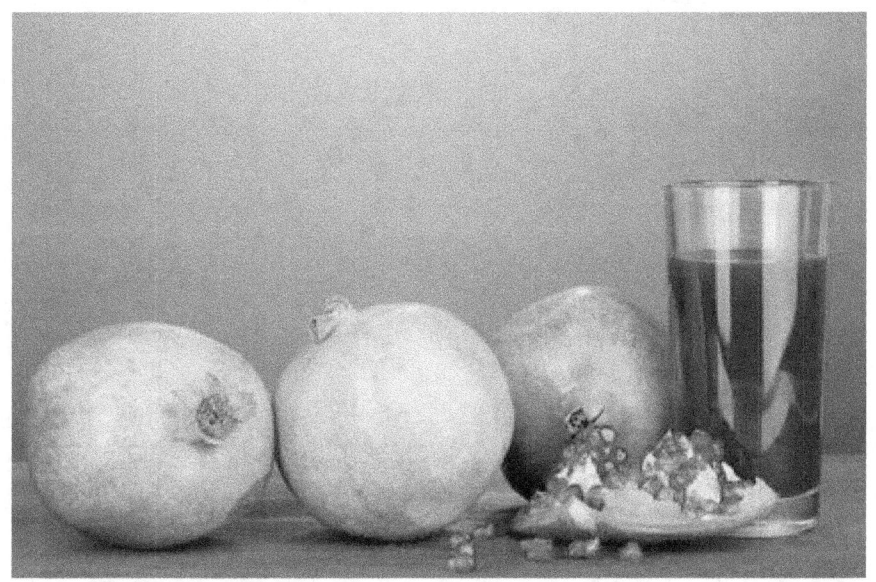

SERVES 2

Cooking Time: 2 minutes

Nutritional Facts: Calories 400, Protein 10 g, Total Fat 4 g, Carbohydrates 89 g

Ingredients

1 small beetroot, peeled

2 pomegranates

3 cups coconut water

2 dates, seeded

Ice cubes

Handful of goji berries

Preparation Method

Combine all the ingredients in a food processor.

Pulse for about a minute, till it becomes a smoothie.

Pour over ice and serve!

Sprout and Pepper Reboot

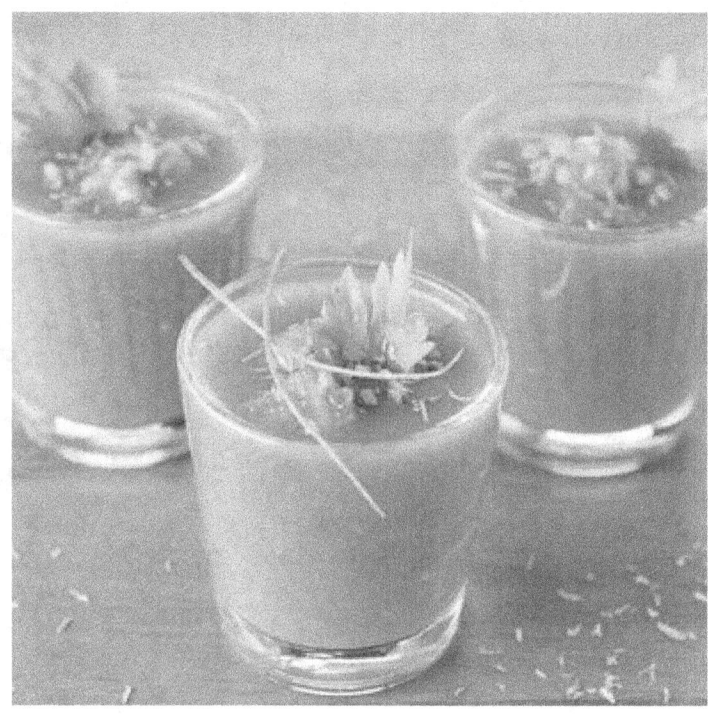

MAKES 2 quarts (about 4 servings)

Cooking Time: 3 minutes

Nutritional Facts: Calories 358, Protein 6.2 g, Total Fat 0.1 g, Carbohydrates 84 g

Ingredients

> 4 red bell peppers, seeded and coarsely diced
>
> 6 kale leaves
>
> 2 lemons, juiced
>
> 4 tomatoes, cut into halves
>
> 4 scallions
>
> Half cup sunflower sprouts
>
> 1 lime, juiced
>
> 4 apples, cored and cut into wedges
>
> Few leaves of fresh oregano

Preparation Method

Except for the lemon and lime juice, pass all the other ingredients through a juicer. Stir to mix.

Pass the juice through a sieve. Discard the residues.

Stir in the lemon and lime juice.

Drink immediately!

Tropical Orange Riser

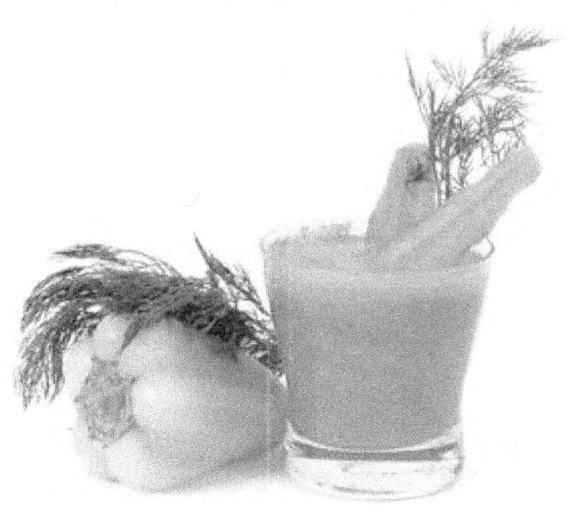

SERVES 2

Cooking Time: 3 minutes

Nutritional Facts: Calories 138, Protein 3 g, Total Fat 0.0 g, Carbohydrates 32 g

Ingredients

> 2 yellow bell peppers, seeded and coarsely diced
>
> 1 green apple, cored and cut into wedges
>
> 2 orange bell peppers, seeded and coarsely diced
>
> 1 lemon, juiced
>
> 2 large carrots

Preparation Method

Except for the lemon juice, pass all the other ingredients through a juicer. Stir to mix.

Pass the juice through a sieve, if required.

Stir in the lemon juice.

Drink immediately!

Peach Pleasure

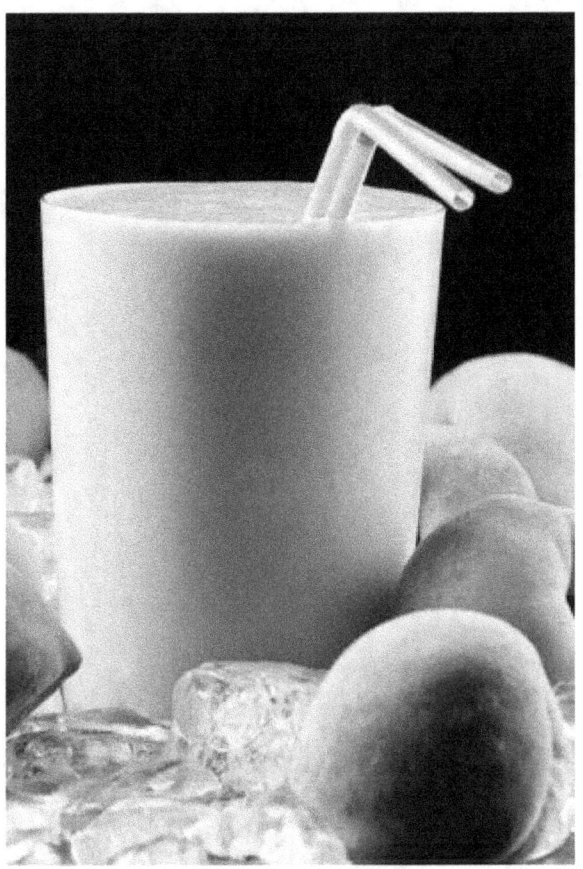

SERVES 2

Cooking Time: 3 minutes

Nutritional Facts: Calories 143, Protein 5 g, Total Fat 0.0 g, Carbohydrates 33 g

Ingredients

> 4 medium carrots
>
> 2 peaches, pitted
>
> 1 (4-inch piece) slice of fresh ginger root
>
> 8 kale leaves

Preparation Method

Juice all the ingredients.

Stir to mix.

Drink immediately!